The
Therapist
Within
YOU

The Therapist Within *You*

A handbook of kinesiology
self-therapy with the pendulum

Jonathan Livingstone

First published in 2009
by Lemniscate Books
43 Clarendon Street, Leamington Spa CV32 4PN, UK
Email info@lemniscatebooks.co.uk

© Jonathan Livingstone 2009

ISBN 978-0-9563179-0-2

British Library Cataloguing in Publication Data.
A catalogue record for this book is available from the British Library.

NOTE:
This book is not intended to replace the guidance of professional health and medical
services. The use of these materials is the responsibility of the user and, although they
are known only to produce benefits and no harm, the author and publisher disclaim any
liability arising from their use. If in doubt, consult your health practitioner.

For Elizabeth and Abigail

Lemniscate Books

Contents

List of Figures

Chapter 18

Foreword by Matthew Thie

You have in your hands a collection of very practical exercises for you to try for yourself. They will develop your self-awareness, release stress, relieve aches and pains, and alleviate other symptoms. The result will be to help you to mobilize your energies to manifest harmony and health and create the life that you want. You will also find here some very fascinating considerations of the nature of consciousness, the unconscious, emotions, and reality.

Jonathan Livingstone provides a concrete and practical approach to empowering individuals to take care of themselves. Very many therapies are done to or for the patient or client; a core principle of energy kinesiology (a main source of the approaches in this book) is that it involves the individual in the process. This means that education, understanding and self-awareness are as important as working on muscles or rubbing acupressure points.

You may or may not agree with Jonathan's philosophical speculations (of course my dog, Max, has consciousness and emotions!); but considering these ideas will go a long way to clarifying your own beliefs about the nature of reality, and may even help you to improve the quality of your perceptions, expand your beliefs, and make your life richer.

Of particular significance here are not just the many suggestions and techniques for accessing and appreciating your emotions, but valuable insights into why you would want to access your emotions, and how to work effectively with them to create the experience of life that you want. Jonathan teaches us practical methods for acknowledging our emotions as friends and allies that serve us. Without proper acknowledgement of our emotions we are not truly living; but, when embraced in a constructive way, they provide the source for a rich, soulful, and fulfilling existence.

In addition to many techniques (much of the Touch for Health system can be accessed in this book), Jonathan brings together his own personal perspective, experiences, and insights. While I have not personally walked myself through all of the exercises in this book (yet!), many involve the same or very similar principles and processes to those I learned in my family, have used throughout my life, and have observed time and again quickly and easily improving how people feel.

A good deal of the material comes from his years of working in the trenches with people who have perhaps a higher than ordinary degree of stress and trauma. His instructions therefore go beyond the basics of everyday balancing, and provide an in-depth and comprehensive guide to applying the pendulum to balancing life energy and tackling issues resulting from stress, confusion and trauma.

Much will be familiar to the practising energy kinesiologist, though it is all presented in a manner that is accessible to the absolute beginner; and Jonathan's fresh personal insights, adaptations and detailed protocol will prove valuable even to the seasoned professional.

Health from within

My parents, John and Carrie Thie, joined together when they were still quite young with the mutual intention of living lives that would somehow contribute to making life better for others, while also taking care of themselves and their family.

My father's focus was chiropractic; my mother's more oriented to psychology. It was my mother's involvement in teaching workshops to lay people in Effective Communication (a programme developed by Tom Gordon, a protégé of Carl Rogers) that formed the model for the workshops that later became known as Touch for Health (TFH). Noting the book's title, *The Therapist Within You*, I am reminded of the early workshops, during the formation of Touch for Health, which were originally called Health from Within. These workshops incorporated elements of George Goodheart's Applied Kinesiology and concepts from Traditional Chinese Medicine in a person-centred, self-responsibility model.

John and Carrie developed the system of Touch for Health to put a set of tools into the hands of everyday people that are deceptively simple yet profoundly effective. Using these tools enhances people's enjoyment of their lives; improves relationships by facilitating mutual support and listening; and enhances health through appropriate, permission-based touch.

In this book, Jonathan Livingstone updates and renews the tradition of looking to our own miraculous internal systems – which include physiology, energy, thoughts and emotions, and which produce both health and disease – to help us to regenerate our bodies and our lives. Although all kinds of external factors can impact on our functioning, all healing comes from within. No healer heals, but rather creates a space, a context, or an opportunity for the internal healing system to function.

The question of self-testing

Involved in the notion of touch in Touch for Health (in addition to touching or rubbing specific body-balancing points) is the idea that another person is taking the time to listen, support and be physically present for your healing and optimum wellness. That's one reason we don't teach self-testing in TFH.

We train people to work with a partner to see which muscles are out of balance and how this might reflect imbalances in their lives – physical, postural, structural, emotional, mental, energetic, dietary, and so on. We also teach people to use an indicator muscle to get clues about what factors might be involved in the individual's symptoms, issues, goals, dreams, desires, stresses and dis-eases.

We don't say that self-testing is no good; we say that it is actually not easy to learn and practice or apply accurately. Indeed, we try to limit muscle testing in TFH to the simplest approach possible that will allow us to balance the physical posture, attitude and life energy flow of the human being. So we avoid asking the body questions or using a muscle test to represent a yes-or-no answer from the body, but rather look for indications of involvement of different energy circuits, or sources of stress, or perhaps just resonance – the presence of 'juice' related to a topic, issue or energy circuit. Then we apply a variety of gentle muscle/energy balancing reflexes to get energy flowing harmoniously.

Experience has shown that it is not easy to self-test reliably enough to balance energy and improve function or, in particular, to identify your own energetic response to foods, ideas, and psychological/emotional issues. Asking questions with muscle testing depends very much on the quality of the question and often reveals more about the bias, beliefs or desires of the tester than any objective truth, and this is amplified in the closed feedback circuit of self-testing. As Jonathan states, muscle testing oneself can take considerable practice and is not readily learned from reading a book.

Nonetheless, this book will help you to navigate the major pitfalls of self-testing, and develop personal references to make the information you gather with the pendulum more concrete and of practical use.

Of primary importance is the fact that any muscle testing reflects the subjective state of an individual, not necessarily any externally verifiable truth. Muscle testing or use of the pendulum is generally considered a lousy way to detect if someone is lying, or if a person is 'good' or 'bad'. It probably won't help you pick any lottery numbers. It is the truth of your body's perceptions and interpretations, of your experience of life; information derived with the pendulum won't stand up in court.

But the pendulum can produce startlingly meaningful clues as to where there is a charge in the system, or where energy is blocked. It can also point to the key issues in a given moment which, when appropriately addressed, will create a shift in energy, posture and attitude that will mobilize the natural internal healing system to create health and vitality.

This book provides a rationale for using the pendulum accurately based on concrete experience, and describes the potential and the limitations of using this instrument. With a better understanding of the workings of muscle testing or using the pendulum you will be in a much better position to:

1   Generate quality information through your testing or checking.
2   Interpret that information in a grounded and practical way.
3   Act on that information in constructive and very profound and powerful ways.
4   Confirm and reinforce the changes and benefits with this bio-feedback and self- awareness tool.

Next steps

There are a plethora of practical tips, instructions, and tools here for approaching your own issues, balancing your energy and moving in the direction of health. Read the ideas presented here and compare them with your own beliefs, accepting and integrating or rejecting the ideas as works for you, and you will significantly increase awareness about your own health and wellbeing. As you actively experience this material you will be able to achieve a new level of self-care, and ways of caring for others.

Even more significantly, you will have a deeper sense and knowledge of the essence of your being, through direct and concrete experience. You will be prepared to live more fully, experience more deeply, and move more whole-heartedly in the direction of your own personal integrity and vitality: to love the life you live, and live the life you love.

You will have a greater understanding and appreciation of the benefits of 'therapy' – psychological, energetic, postural, perhaps even medical – and thus be able to take a far more active role in your own therapy and personal development. You will also be able to recognize and reinforce the benefits of continuing therapy with professionals and experts, if this is necessary, as well as with respect to your own ongoing self-care and self-therapy.

You may find that simply applying a few favourite balancing exercises from this book is all you want or need at present to make your life just a bit better. Or you may find that you have enjoyed some or all of the exercises, and are hungry for more; or that you are hungry for some fellowship and/or support and instruction to increase your effectiveness with these techniques. I highly recommend that you reach out to others to practise these skills, and amplify these experiences.

There are many formal workshops available in the UK and throughout the world. Of course, from my perspective as head of Touch for Health Education, Touch for Health forms a core, foundational programme. Many – but far from all – of the TFH techniques are incorporated into this book. If you would like direct instruction, demonstration and hands-on, guided practice with fellow participants, that will deepen your understanding, strengthen your skills, and enhance your effectiveness, then I urge you to enrol on a TFH workshop. Check the information on pages 333–4 at the end of this book for information on training.

Each one teach one

Once you have done the reading, reflecting, private experiencing, practis-ing and sharing with others, you will be ready to pass on the flame. Your personal comprehension and effectiveness will increase exponentially if you endeavour to share these techniques with other people. And if you can teach one other person, why not teach ten? If ten, why not 100? TFH has spread from one chiropractor in California to hundreds of lay instructors throughout the world. Currently there are over 30 trainers of instructors in 25 different countries, and TFH has benefited perhaps millions of people since its launch in 1973.

Part of the beauty of this work is that it attracts to it the people who can most benefit, and people with a natural healing gift. You too are a seed that can multiply and ultimately benefit millions. You can begin the process through sharing this work with family and friends; by incorporating the techniques into your therapeutic/health care practice; or by becoming a formal instructor of TFH or kinesiology practitioner. Readers in Britain may be interested in learning more about the Professional TFH Practitioner Training in England which is the only training of its kind in the world.

An enriching Journey

In this diverse and personal work, Jonathan presents us with a wealth of ideas, a lot of practical information, and invitations to experiences that can profoundly affect the ways that we perceive and experience our lives. Take the journey and try on these concepts and ideas. Specifically, try out the exercises. This alone will do a lot to enhance your sense of your own reality and actually improve the quality of your experience of life.

We all know that riches – whether in material form or personal qualities – in themselves do not equate to happiness or satisfaction in life. Rather, the extent to which we utilize our resources to allow ourselves the opportunity to have a full, soulful experience and appreciation of life is the extent to which our riches are of real value. In that light, consider the book in your hands to be the kind of gold that will enable you to envision and create the life you wish.

Matthew Thie
Echo Park, Los Angeles
November 2008

Matthew Thie is Head of Touch for Health Education and Director of Research for the International Kinesiology College

Preliminaries

The first principle of the new therapy is self-responsibility. The reader assumes full responsibility for the use of the material in this book. Although these methods are safe and are not known to cause any harm but only good, the author cannot accept any liability for any negative consequences arising from their use. Sometimes, starting to work meaningfully on yourself involves stirring up your emotional pot so that very uncomfortable emotions come to the surface. Should you experience this, difficult though it is, you have an opportunity to finally resolve the issues that underlie them. The perpetual subjugation of those emotions is maintained at a cost. I strongly recommend that you keep working on your issues until they are processed and you feel better. You will not only feel better, you will be profoundly healed. However, you may need more support than a book can provide. If in any doubt, the guidance of a qualified therapist or medical doctor is advised.

Preface

Everybody wants to be physically and emotionally healthy. There is no shortage of advice and books on all aspects of health, including nutrition, self-help techniques and remedies of all kinds. But which is the best advice for you? You know that health is a complex matter. Good health requires not only exercise and good food, but also relates to lifestyle, stress levels, emotional intelligence, beliefs and past traumas. And everybody is different. What are the most effective things you can do to get healthy and remain healthy?

This book aims to answer these questions. Primarily, not by giving advice, but by showing you how to make the best choices for yourself. The best advice comes not from proclaimed experts but from your own body. Your body knows what its problems are and how to remedy them. You just need to gain access to that knowledge.

The pendulum and the discipline of kinesiology provide this access. Learning to use a pendulum is easy. Achieving consistent and reliable results and determining the optimum answers requires the principles of kinesiology. Adapting kinesiology techniques to the pendulum helps turn the pendulum from a crude and temperamental tool into a precision psycho-surgical instrument.

Kinesiology makes available countless techniques to balance your energies, improve your health, heal past traumas and resolve present problems, in collaboration with the knowledge and wisdom of the therapist within you – your body.

Not only will you be shown how to get reliable information from your body, you will learn a wide variety of highly effective tried-and-tested treatments (called *corrections* in kinesiology) to help your body heal itself and function optimally. You are not even confined to the techniques presented here: any other healing modalities that you know or learn can be incorporated and included in your repertoire of remedies.

This book will teach you:

- How to identify problems.
- Where problems come from and how they develop.
- How to formulate effective and achievable goals.
- How to apply some of the most effective contemporary therapeutic techniques.
- How to resolve your problems, not only in their present manifestation but also at their source.

You will learn how to use the pendulum as a surrogate for another person, enabling you to help others. If you have children, or other family members willing to accept your help, the methods in this book will teach you how to help them resolve their problems, improve their learning, remove blocks to their development and maintain their optimum health – in exactly the same way as you would work on your own issues.

You will also, I hope, find a coherent account of the nature and origins of therapeutic problems. The truth is that emotional issues are no longer a mystery. Although it has taken over a century for the pieces to have been found, they do fit together to form a coherent picture. My intention is to present this picture to you more clearly, perhaps, than can be found anywhere else.

Therapeutic techniques are carefully explained, and there are exercises to help you to understand and apply them. You will learn:

1. To apply a wide range of highly effective kinesiology corrections and other methods, including EFT, to yourself. These will form a therapeutic reservoir of techniques to help you resolve virtually any problem.
2. A comprehensive protocol to address and resolve emotional and emotion-related issues – which will be like having your own personal therapist always available to you.
3. How to test foods, supplements, essences and other remedies to determine those that will serve you the best.

Reliable access to the wisdom of your unconscious body means you're not reliant on guesswork or the prejudices of conscious thinking (or, worse, trust in an unknown person or method), as your body is able to choose the best path for you. Through the pendulum, your body will tell you:

○   What the priority problem exactly is.

○   Where it comes from.

○   The best way to remedy it.

You may be able to help yourself – in consultation with your medical doctor, of course – reduce and terminate medication; and give yourself alternatives to drugs which, although effective in alleviating symptoms, do not resolve the problem itself and often cause physiological harm. By finding and resolving the (emotional) sources of your physical ailments, the physical ailments are usually able to heal automatically.

Here is a wonderful tool for health and life: it is the new self-healing; the therapy for the twenty-first century. You will be able to find out everything you need to know to improve your health and achieve your goals – all determined by the one that knows you and knows what's best for you better than anyone else possibly can: your own body.

A word of caution. Kinesiology with the pendulum does not provide a means to diagnose illnesses. Leave that to the medical doctors. Kinesiology is a holistic practice. The concern of kinesiology is not to diagnose or treat symptoms but to resolve the sources of problems and bring the whole body into balance and health. This is the best and safest way to heal, maintain health, prevent disease, resolve problems, achieve goals, assure happiness, and bring you back to your authentic self.

Acknowledgements

Thanks in particular to my wife, Elizabeth, without whose active encouragement this book would still be just a very good idea. Thanks to Julianne Miller for her advice on an early draft, and to Rita Sharkey, a great friend and a brilliant kinesiologist, for her nurturing faith in my kinesiology.

Thank you to the highly accomplished singer and dancer (and West End star) Leyla Pellegrini and the actor Jumaan Short for being models for the figures. Thank you to Sebastian Parsons, CEO of Elysia, for providing studio facilities for the photographs.

I also owe much to my trainers, including Daphne Clarke, my Three In One Concepts trainer, and Sandy Gannon, whose dedication to Touch for Health has galvanized me and energized kinesiology on this European island; to my students, from whom I'm constantly learning; and to my clients, whose courage and commitment are a constant source of inspiration.

I am greatly indebted to a few innovative thinkers on whom much of the material in this book is directly based. Primarily: the late Dr John Thie, who created Touch for Health – a kinesiology system for non-medically trained people derived from the late Dr George Goodheart's pioneering work in what became Applied Kinesiology[1] – and his son Matthew Thie, an inspiration to all Touch for Healthers, who is dedicated to continuing his father's work.

I am also grateful to the late Gordon Stokes and Daniel Whiteside, co-founders of Three In One Concepts, Inc., a worldwide recognized educational corporation, who have kindly permitted me to include a number of corrections (see chapter 14). This permission was given even though self-therapy using a pendulum is not recognized by them nor is pendulum therapy any part of their trademarked 'One Brain' system.

To Dr Edward Bach, the medical doctor who recognized the role of the spiritual and of personality in health and pioneered the use of flower remedies to treat emotional states, I am grateful for his descriptions of his remedies, reproduced in chapter 18.

Kinesiology has given rise to new energy therapies that don't require muscle testing, notably Emotional Freedom Techniques, developed and promoted by Gary Craig. His system provides a vital tool in this text.

I am grateful to Dr Charles Krebs for his kind permission to reproduce the modified Ridler nutrition chart.

There are numerous other practitioners and thinkers whose work has provided conscious and unconscious illumination for the ideas presented here. Their contributions inform this work. The errors are, of course, solely my own.

---

1   Applied Kinesiology (AK) was further developed and codified by the Goodheart Study Group Leaders who later formed the International College of Applied Kinesiology (ICAK). The Touch for Health lay training programme, created by Dr John Thie, was established at the same time as the ICAK was formed. The sharing of both of these models (AK for licensed professionals; TFH for lay people and instructors) resulted in the general field of work using muscle testing together with the energetic and holistic model of healing and wellness which has come to be called *energy kinesiology*.

Introduction

The heart of this book is about kinesiology: a fascinating, complex, mis-understood and generally little-known therapy. But kinesiology is one of the most sophisticated, effective and adaptable non-medical healing systems ever developed. What's more, any therapy can be incorporated into kinesi-ology, which makes it infinitely flexible. As well as kinesiology, a number of particularly useful methods from other contemporary disciplines (such as NLP and EFT) are made available for you in this text. The aim is to give you the best possible tools for self-healing that can be learned from a book.

The techniques you will learn are highly effective and powerful. Thousands of kinesiologists and their clients attest to the healing capability of these methods. Procedures from kinesiology are being used successfully by doctors, homoeopaths, chiropractors and osteopaths, as well as kinesiologists, in countries all over the world. They are also used increasingly in schools. If your child is drawing lazy eights (lemniscates), massaging specific reflex points and being encouraged to drink good quantities of mineral water at school there's a kinesiologist at work.

What can kinesiology help?

Kinesiology is known to help a whole range of physical and emotional ail-ments. By bringing the body back into balance (see chapter 9, The Energy of Everything) kinesiology (and its incorporated therapies) can help just about any therapeutic problem. Kinesiology can balance the body in the present, providing a temporary remedy to the problem; and it will also let you find the sources of a problem and find the best ways to resolve them.

It's not always immediately clear whether a physical ailment has an emo-tional cause or not. The medical profession (certainly in the UK) is generally unaware of the emotional sources of problems (although this is beginning to change), often inappropriately attributing genetic causes. This happens often, for example, when people present with a weight or eating problem. Medical doctors generally have little understanding of the emotional causes underlying physical manifestations. Even psychiatrists generally treat emotional problems with drugs rather than identifying and resolving the issues themselves.

If doctors can't find a physical problem, you can be pretty confident there's an emotional issue to be resolved. But emotional issues are also often key (but not necessarily causal) factors in apparently more strictly physical illnesses as well. Indeed, any physical ailment or disease can have an emotional contributor or aspect. Resolving the sources of a problem and balancing the body make physical healing possible.

Healing is natural; it's always the body that heals itself. If the body is given appropriate opportunities to heal itself, it will do so. Everyone knows that a physical injury needs time and opportunity to heal. If a physical injury is not given this opportunity it will not heal properly. And if you keep doing the thing that led to the physical ailment, the problem is likely to be exacerbated. Exactly the same is true of emotional wounds – which are the causes of subsequent therapeutic problems. Kinesiology (like other effective therapies) provides the body appropriate opportunities to heal these emotional wounds, thereby resolving the therapeutic problem.[1]

Using the techniques presented here I have helped individuals to resolve a huge variety of problems and clear obstacles to the achievement of goals. Thousands of other therapists have used similar techniques successfully with clients. You will be able to help yourself to heal, develop, or change. Just take the trouble to work through the book carefully and do the exercises. It doesn't matter what issues you want to deal with – increasing your motivation; overcoming insomnia; getting off (prescribed, legal or illegal) drugs;[2] improving your confidence; healing your digestive problems; clearing blocks to happiness; resolving emotional traumas; improving relationships; healing serious illness; reducing stress; overcoming anxiety or fears;

---

1   Just talking about it is rarely enough.

2   Consulting your medical doctor is necessary before changing medication. The guidance of a therapist and support group is strongly recommended for drug and alcohol addiction.

depression; or anything else – these techniques will almost certainly help, possibly dramatically.

As you work through the exercises, methods and corrections you will prob-ably find yourself becoming less upset, tired, angry, depressed, and more energized, relaxed, motivated, healthy and happy – and self-aware.

Working with kinesiology

Kinesiology is a holistic system of natural health care which addresses all four dimensions of being: emotional, structural, biochemical and spiritual. Its primary tool is muscle monitoring (generally called muscle testing), which is a means of deriving responses from the body in relation to verbal or non-verbal stimuli presented to the body.

You'll be using a pendulum rather than muscle monitoring; but it will be use-ful to understand how muscle monitoring works, since many of the methods you will learn derive from this discipline.

Muscle monitoring is a bio-feedback process whereby information about the body is communicated through a muscle. The body is presented with a stimu-lus, question or challenge (verbal or non-verbal) and, in response, the muscle being monitored responds by holding or giving way.

For example, the client stretches his or her arm out to the side and, after the introduction of a stimulus, the tester or therapist gently and steadily pushes down on the arm, just above the wrist. The deltoid (shoulder) muscle will either lock the arm in place easily, or the muscle will not lock and the arm will be pressed downward.

In kinesiology the stimulus may be in the form of a verbal question, a thought, a memory brought back into awareness, or a substance put on or close to the body. The following are examples of stressors which produce an unlocking muscle:

  o   recalling a painful or traumatic experience;
  o   thinking of performing a difficult task;
  o   putting a mobile phone to the ear;
  o   putting a food you are sensitive or allergic to on the navel (or in the mouth).

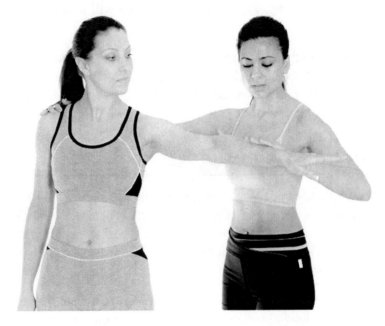

(a) Muscle locking

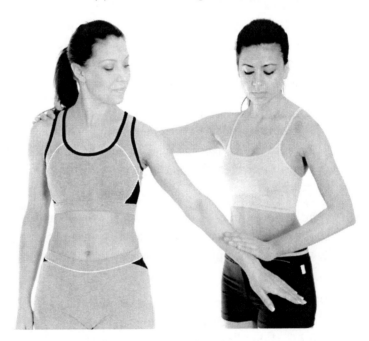

(b) Muscle unlocking

Figure 0.1 Muscle monitoring

Thinking of anything that stresses you will make a locked muscle unlock, even when you are not consciously aware of the stress. Kinesiology is therefore the ideal therapy for discovering exactly the factors which stress the body.

When the body is under stress its resources are being strained, and this is detrimental to the body. The body is designed to cope with moderate amounts of stress; but when stress is severe or long lasting, the body suffers damage.

When tested, a muscle unlocks when:

- A stimulus is introduced that is stressful to the body.[3]
- The body gives a NO response to a question or statement.

A muscle remains locked when:

- A stimulus is introduced that is not stressful (such as a happy or neutral thought; a benign substance) or is beneficial to the body.
- The body gives a YES response to a question or statement.

A muscle which is unlocked due to stress will lock when:

- A stimulus is introduced which helps to resolve or counter the stress.

In this way the body communicates information through the response of the muscle. From muscle monitoring it is easy to establish:

1. Whether a stimulus is beneficial or harmful to the body.
2. Whether a stimulus can directly help a specific problem (by locking an unlocked muscle).
3. Yes or no answers to questions or statements.

This is just scratching the surface of what is possible with kinesiology. You may already be beginning to glimpse some of the applications of muscle testing.

---

3   However, a stimulus can be so stressful that the muscle seizes up and remains locked. This is a common condition which I call hyperstress. The kinesiologist should always be prepared to test for this possibility or a hyperstressed response will be overlooked. For more on hyperstress, see below (pre-test # 7).

There is one obvious disadvantage kinesiology has when it comes to self-help: it is very difficult to muscle test oneself. It is possible, and many people do it, but it can take considerable practice and is not readily learnt from a book.

Because of this (not helped that alternative healing has been disparaged by the medical establishment) there are not many kinesiology self-help books. So this powerful and effective healing modality has remained little recognized and under-utilized.

Using a pendulum allows all the body's information to be accessible to you without assistance and without muscle testing. This makes the wonderful system of kinesiology available as a comprehensive self-help tool. With a pendulum you can do the equivalent of a muscle test for yourself. In kinesiology (to reiterate) a holding muscle means YES/POSITIVE, and an unlocking muscle means NO/STRESSED. In similar fashion, the pendulum swings in one direction for YES/POSITIVE, and swings in another direction for NO/STRESSED.

Imagine the benefits of being able to use this practice in everyday life. Using the pendulum for self-kinesiology, you will, for example, be able to:

- Identify environmental stressors.
- Identify emotional stressors.
- Identify the sources of your issues.
- Identify the best remedy for any problem.
- Identify the best approaches to resolve any issue.
- Identify and avoid foods that you are sensitive or allergic to.
- Identify nutritional deficiencies.
- Choose the most beneficial of a choice of supplements.

This information, and the protocols, approaches and techniques in this book will enable you to do self-therapy in a way that's never been possible before.

Responses to a stimulus

One way the kinesiologist elicits information from the body is by using verbal questions or statements. The unconscious body perfectly understands language. However, when asking verbal questions there is a danger that the questions will be unclear or ambiguous, because wording questions precisely is tricky. When using the pendulum it is therefore important to be vigilant: choose your words carefully and take great care in the formulation of sentences. You need to be very clear that you know precisely what you are asking. Only ask those things that are within the remit of your body to answer.

The kinesiologist also elicits information from the body using non-verbal means, such as placing vials containing a substance (such as a food or remedy) close to the body (on the navel, for example), or by touching specific points on the body. These methods address the body energetically, without the medium of language.

Some kinesiologists prefer the non-verbal approach since it seems to be a more direct way of communicating with the body. However, eliciting information non-verbally also has difficulties. When a vial is placed close to the body, the body may not be able to 'read' it unless the content of the vial is a high-energy substance.[4] When the substance is not high energy, the body may respond more to your intention than to the contents of the vial. Generally, this is fine – in fact, it's very helpful. An intention is equivalent to a verbal statement or question.

The pendulum – how reliable an instrument?

The pendulum is an ancient instrument. In the mid-nineteenth century – at a time when it was widely used to tell the sex of an unborn child – the French chemist Michel Eugene Chevreul (1786–1889) demonstrated scientifically that the pendulum was communicating unconscious knowledge. Today the pendulum is often called Chevreul's pendulum and is used in clinical hypnosis – as well as in more esoteric circles.

The major difficulty with the pendulum, however, is that – as people very often report – it can give inconsistent, unreliable and even completely nonsensical responses. This leads many people who learn to use the pendulum with initial enthusiasm to give it up disillusioned. I had the same experience many years ago and put it away – before I encountered kinesiology.

---

4   High-energy substances include homeopathic remedies and flower essences.

The three primary factors that lead to erroneous muscle testing results are stress, conscious desire interference and lack of permission. These factors can also affect the pendulum.

Stress

Some forms of stress can interfere with the body's energy circuits and produce false muscle tests.[5] Kinesiology recognizes that muscle monitoring can give anomalous responses unless these problems are checked for and, if necessary, corrected. By using kinesiology procedures you will ensure that the pendulum gives correct and accurate readings despite the effects of stress.

Conscious desire

The pendulum gives us unconscious information. That is the point of it. But *conscious* desires and expectations can override the expression of the unconscious body and instead of getting information from the body we end up getting the response of the conscious mind. When desires get in the way, the pendulum doesn't give an honest answer but the answer we consciously desire.

This makes sense: the unconscious is at the service of the conscious mind. The conscious mind can overrule the unconscious in most circumstances (except perhaps those involving physical danger or great emotional threat). For example, you may once have wanted to establish a relationship with someone (or make a decision) in contradiction to your body, which was giving you palpable somatic feelings (maybe a heaviness in your abdomen) to stay away. You are probably willing to acknowledge now that your unconscious was right, you should have stayed away; but, at the time, your conscious mind pulled rank and you foolishly pursued the relationship. Willpower is precisely this: overruling the preferences of the unconscious or body – the unconscious body[6] – to do what the conscious mind insists on.

---

5   Such stress can lead to what's called switching or central meridian over-energy. More on these later.

6   The word unconscious is very often found in the collocation unconscious mind, which we learned from Freud. This conception has proved an obstacle to a proper understanding of the relationship of conscious and unconscious. We tend to think of the psyche as referring to the mind; in fact, it means soul (linking it inextricably to feeling). Psychology should relate to the body and not simply to the narrow concept of 'mind'. The conception of the unconscious presented here

You will learn a technique, introduced in print here for the first time, that helps prevent the conscious mind from overruling the information transmitted from the unconscious body. Using this technique, which I call the *pendulum mode*, the unconscious body is able to express its real intentions in spite of the preferences of the conscious mind.

Permission

The third major reason that people often encounter anomalous responses from the pendulum is the unconscious rejection of the issue. There are some things your body isn't prepared to make available to the conscious mind. When this is the case, it doesn't matter whether you are using hypnosis, muscle testing or a pendulum – the body isn't going to spill the beans.

If, for example, there is one period of your life that you have little conscious recollection of, you may justifiably suspect that severe trauma occurred during that time.[7] Amnesia is not arbitrary; and in all probability there is no damage to the part of the brain associated with that memory. Your unconscious has been keeping the memories from you for good reason. You shouldn't expect your unconscious suddenly to let you know what happened because you're swinging a pendulum about (just as it wouldn't if you were in hypnotic trance). But there are ways of accessing that information. This is an important issue that will be addressed in various ways in the coming chapters.

In short: *you need permission from your unconscious for whatever work you do with the pendulum.*

---

is radically different from Freud's unconscious mind. The concept of conscious mind makes sense; it is the mind – thoughts – that are experienced as conscious. But the notion of unconscious mind is unhelpful and inaccurate. I refer to *unconscious body*, and when I use the term unconscious, it should be understood that I am referring to the unconscious body not 'mind'.

7   Trauma is often associated with experiences of marked severity. In this text it is used to refer to any experience which has not been satisfactorily resolved and still carries an emotional charge in the body. Such unresolved experiences are significant because they continue to determine how a person responds to events – usually without any conscious awareness. I think it's highly probable that unresolved traumas also continue to stress the body, even when the person has no conscious awareness of the incident or does not acknowledge the feelings it gives rise to.

By the way, the pendulum will give an answer to anything you ask (as will muscle testing). It will tell you next week's winning lottery numbers and the size of the universe. But this doesn't mean the answer is true or accurate – as you can readily establish (at least with regard to next week's numbers).

A philosophy of healing

The pendulum provides a way for your unconscious to communicate directly with your conscious mind and, through its abundant wisdom, let you know what it wants for your health and development.

Is the unconscious really so wise? And why is it so useful to get information from your unconscious? According to Milton Erickson, the father of modern hypnotherapy, people go for therapy for one reason only: their conscious mind is out of rapport with their unconscious. Put another way, becoming stressed or ill is a result of your conscious mind losing touch with what your body wants and needs. When you need therapy or healing, it is because your conscious mind is disconnected from your feelings (the communications of your unconscious body). If you had remained in tune with your body, it's likely that you wouldn't have become stressed or ill.

Your body knows what's good for it. By its very nature, your body will look after, protect and nurture itself. That is how it is constituted. The body knows what nutrients it needs. It knows what gives pleasure and happiness. Left to its own devices – without interference – the body would take absolute care of itself. Animals do this entirely unconsciously. They don't need a conscious mind to survive – which is just as well, since they don't have one.

But human beings have the capacity to interfere with this natural process. Your body communicates its wishes[8] (primarily) through feelings, but your conscious mind can readily override your unconscious body as you suppress or deny your feelings. This allows you to do things detrimental to your health and happiness. It can be handy, useful and fun to go against your body's impulses in specific circumstances.

---

8 Of course the unconscious doesn't literally have wishes, since a wish is an expression of a conscious mind; but the unconscious does strive for what's best for the person.

However, in general, going against and suppressing your feelings is done at great cost. If you do this for long enough you're in danger of losing touch with certain feelings altogether (as smokers and other drug takers often do). This creates a division between your conscious identity on the one side and, on the other, who you really are and who you are meant to be. Your conscious mind is out of rapport with your unconscious body and you're not happy or congruent.

Now you are at odds with yourself. The uncomfortable feelings, trapped inside the body, are probably increasing in intensity – the more they are ignored the more they strive to find expression.[9] They won't rest until you have properly faced and resolved them. Depending on your experience and how you are constituted, this expression will be through emotional distress of some kind or through physical illness, or both. Ignoring or suppressing your feelings can have disastrous consequences for your health.

Some people do everything they can to hold the troublesome feelings inside and deny them expression, creating massive internal stress. Others give them expression by directing them outwards on to unsuspecting others. The psychological basis of inappropriate aggression is the suppression and displacement of anger. It can express itself in enjoyment of violent movies, books or games, or support for war – which provide an outlet and temporary relief but never a resolution or healing.

There are people who externalize their pain on to others; and there are people who internalize their pain within themselves (this is clearly a generalization since everyone to a certain extent does both). People who are interested in self-help or therapy tend to be internalizers. People who blame other people for their troubles are highly unlikely to pursue therapy or real personal development since they are the blamers – which means it's not their fault. Blamers even externalize their self-doubt so that they are the paradigm of certainty.

Since you are working on yourself, you are highly likely generally to intern-alize rather than externalize. That makes you much less of a danger to society (or indeed to other societies) – if that's any consolation – but more of a danger directly to yourself. Not for much longer!

---

9   Freud calls this *the return of the repressed*.

Ill health – spiritual, emotional, and to a great extent physical[10] – is a consequence of the unresolved traumas held in the body. Depending on their severity and complexity, and how tightly the lid is kept closed, the emotion in these traumas leaks or crashes into our daily lives through our behaviour in response to specific triggers. Fortunately, we don't need to suffer in silence or thunder; we can get help and we can help ourselves.

Emotional healing

Healing is best achieved by addressing and resolving the traumas from the past that prevent you from being yourself, trap you with problems, and hinder you from moving towards your goals. Feelings associated with these unresolved traumas underlie the inappropriate and undesired behaviours that constitute problems.

Feelings, too often marginalized and subordinated to reason and conscious thought, in fact motivate all behaviour. People act in the way that they do primarily because of feelings, not thoughts. Thoughts provide the rationale, the justification; feelings are the true instigators.

Issues therefore relate to feelings, not thoughts. If your problems related simply to thoughts you could easily change them with an act of will – after all, you are mostly in control of your thoughts, aren't you? Thoughts are the constituents of the conscious mind. Without the conscious mind there are no thoughts; and without thoughts there is no conscious mind.[11]

We have conscious control over our thoughts and behaviour, but we do not have conscious control over our feelings. By denying our feelings, far from banishing them from the body, we simply drive them underground, where they have more power over us because we don't know that they're there or what they're doing. We live healthily by acknowledging our feelings and responding appropriately to them – rather than ignoring, denying or suppressing them.

---

10   The link between physical illness and emotional issues has been increasingly recognized even by practitioners of traditional medicine with the advances in psychoneuroimmunology.

11   Persistent, unwanted or obsessive thoughts are actually generated by unacknowledged or denied feelings.

Most people are out of touch with at least some of their important feelings. Kinesiology, through the pendulum, can bring you back into contact with your feelings, your needs and your true self – freeing you from the limiting constraints you have adopted as a result of your upbringing and the collective beliefs of society.

The body is crying out to express its wishes. Of course, unless we are at the edge of our senses (and in danger of taking leave of them), it's not going to communicate with us in words. If you hear voices, you have good reason to be concerned. The medium of the body is feelings; that is, somatic, physical sensations.[12] It's helpful that the body's medium of expression is distinct from that of the conscious mind. In proportion to the extent to which you get in touch with your feelings, acknowledge them and respond appropriately to them, in that proportion are you healthy and have the foundations for happiness.

The pendulum is the tool to facilitate this communication between unconscious body and conscious mind, and kinesiology provides numerous methods to heal traumas and restore balance. This book teaches powerful techniques from kinesiology and other contemporary therapies to improve health and promote internal peace and happiness, providing a framework to do self-therapy in a systematic way.

Part I introduces the pendulum and explains how to use it. You will learn the initial checks required to ensure the pendulum gives you accurate and reliable information from your unconscious. You will be introduced to essential kinesiology techniques and learn how to be a surrogate for others. At the end of part 1 you will be able to give yourself and others therapy (called a *balance* in kinesiology) using the tools learned so far.

Part II begins with a brief description of how human consciousness evolved, and how problems are created, sustained and manifest themselves. This is followed by a brief account of the concept of qi and the body's energy channels. An understanding of energy and the channels, deriving from traditional Chinese medicine, is not a requirement to use the methods presented here. However, since these concepts lie at the heart of kinesiology, I think it's helpful to know something about how they are conceptualized.

---

12   The unconscious communicates in other subtle ways too, such as through an inkling of something, or making us notice something in our environment; and through what Freud called *parapraxes* (Freudian slips).

You will be taught how to determine which energy channels are under-energized or over-energized. You will learn fundamental kinesiology corrections to assist the lymphatic system and the vascular system, and other techniques to bring your body (and your energy system) back into balance. These techniques will improve your posture and physiological functions, and will encourage physical and emotional health and well-being. They will also often be required to resolve specific emotional issues.

The last few chapters in part II will help you to assess where you are right now and identify your issues. You will learn how to formulate and word your goals. By the end of part II you will know the procedure to carry out a full kinesiology balance for yourself.

Part III introduces a further collection of extremely effective kinesiology techniques. You will also learn about the effect of various environmental factors and how to identify and (where ecological in terms of your system) overcome allergies and sensitivities.

In this section you will discover how to use the highly effective energy therapy called Emotional Freedom Techniques (EFT). EFT, a powerful tool for self-healing in itself, becomes even more effective when combined with the pendulum. EFT with the pendulum will help you to overcome past traumas and the outdated strategies and limiting beliefs deriving from them.

You will learn how to test for nutritional deficiencies, and whether specific foods are benefiting you or otherwise – including identifying and, where applicable, resolving food sensitivities and allergies. Finally, you will find out how to identify the most beneficial supplements and remedies and their optimum doses.

The chapters of this book are intended to be read consecutively. Information in later pages depends on an understanding of principles and procedures outlined in earlier pages. Certainly, part I should be studied carefully before working with the techniques in other chapters.

I recommend that you do all the exercises as you come upon them. Don't just read them. By doing the exercises you are not only improving the health of your whole being, you are giving your unconscious the opportunity to learn about them, how they work, and what their effects are. Doing this will greatly help your body's understanding of this energy work. By giving your body a chance to understand the processes, the responses you get from the pendulum will become very reliable. If you try to use the text as a reference book without doing the exercises your body may not know which exercises are the most helpful. The exercises are relatively brief. If they take longer, it is probably because they are of particular importance to you. The same is probably true of any exercises you want to avoid.

There is a lot of information in the pages that follow. My intention is to be as comprehensive as possible without overwhelming you. Occasionally, where the information is in danger of going beyond this threshold, I have provided warning symbols in the margin. The symbol A§ in the left margin represents the beginning of such material; its appearance in the right margin signifies its end. This material can be skipped during a first reading should your mind begin to boggle.

Remember, these techniques are going to help you to heal and will almost certainly transform you. You may be bewildered that they are not more widely known or that it has taken you this time to discover them. There are secrets here to share with the world; the more that people achieve peace within themselves, the less harm they do to others. With enhanced emotional health, relationships improve and we help to create a better world.

But healing is a challenge – to yourself, first; and then to everyone else around you. You will cease to accept bad treatment and lack of respect. You will no longer put up with unsatisfactory circumstances. You will be regarded differently. Your friends may change; or you may change your friends. The world is going to be different. You are going to be different. It's not going to be easy, but it is going to be worth it. I invite you to take up the challenge.

Part I
CONNECTING WITH THE BODY

1
Contacting
the Therapist Within

The pendulum is your route into the wisdom of the body. It allows your body to communicate with you.

You are going to use kinesiology principles with the pendulum to make sure that the information you receive is reliable and accurate. For this reason, although your tool will be the pendulum rather than muscle testing, it is useful to have an understanding of how muscle testing works.

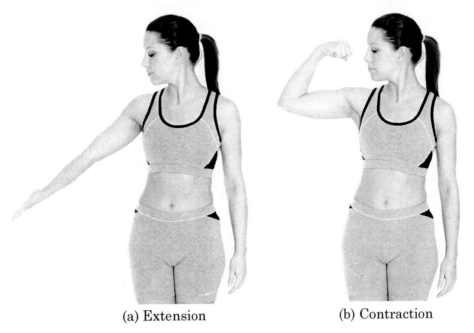

(a) Extension   (b) Contraction

Figure 1.1 The biceps in extension and contraction

Here is a brief and oversimplified explanation. The postural muscles stretch from one bone (the origin of the muscle) to another bone (the insertion of the muscle), passing through a joint. When a muscle is contracted, or shortened, the insertion of the muscle is pulled closer to the origin. For example, in flexing (bending) the arm (with the palm facing the shoulder) you contract the biceps and bring the insertion of the muscle (top of forearm) closer to the origin (shoulder) (see figure 1.1). In a muscle test the muscle is partially contracted (the insertion is pulled closer to the origin); it is then tested as gentle pressure is applied to move the insertion away from the origin of the muscle (to extend it). If the muscle can hold easily and locks, the circuit is in tact. If the muscle unlocks and the limb is unable to hold, there is an imbalance in the circuit.

In kinesiology there are two main ways of using a muscle to obtain information from the body. The first is where a muscle is used as a *general indicator* – as described in the introduction – to answer yes-or-no questions or reveal the body's stressed or unstressed response to a stimulus. The second is where an individual muscle is tested to find imbalances in the specific energy circuit that relates to that muscle. For example the psoas muscle is tested to register imbalances in the kidney circuit.

You will be using the pendulum exclusively as a general indicator. Rather than monitoring whether a muscle locks (unstressed) or does not lock (stressed), you will be looking at the swing of the pendulum. Whether the pendulum's response is YES/POSITIVE or NO/STRESSED the arm has to move to make the pendulum swing. For YES/POSITIVE the pendulum moves in one direction; for NO/STRESSED it moves in another direction. Both YES/POSITIVE and NO/STRESSED require a similar, unconscious and virtually imperceptible, exertion of the body.

Pendulum principles

The principle of the pendulum is simple. Verbally or otherwise you ask the unconscious body questions or give it challenges and the body responds by subtly moving the arm, allowing the pendulum to swing in one direction or another. The pendulum exaggerates the arm's subtle movement and provides a means of seeing it as if magnified. In this way the unconscious can communicate directly with you. The principle is equivalent to using the general indicator muscle in kinesiology, or using ideo-motor responses in hypnosis.[1]

First of all you're going to need a pendulum to use – but you'd probably guessed that already. A pendulum designed specifically for the purpose is ideal because it is crafted to be particularly responsive to the smallest muscle movements. However, the choice of pendulum isn't of great import-ance. Some people are keen that you don't touch their pendulum. That's up to them, of course. Your energy on their pendulum or their energy on your pendulum makes no difference to its swing.

You need something that swings readily. It's no more complicated than that. It could be a crystal at the end of a chain, for example. You don't want a chain that is too long or it takes time for it to change its direction of movement. And you don't want it to be too short or it takes too much effort to get it moving. Similarly with weight. Too heavy and it requires too much energy to move it. But it needs to be heavy enough to register movement.

There's no point in simply reading this: have your pendulum to hand!

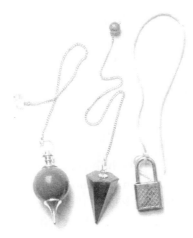

Figure 1.2 Pendulums

---

1   An ideo-motor response is elicited during hypnosis to signal an unconscious response to a question. For example, the unconscious body lifts one finger for yes and another finger for no, with no conscious involvement.

Activating the pendulum

Now that you are in possession of your pendulum, hold the chain (or string) between your thumb and forefinger, and check that it can swing freely in all different directions without changing your grip. It should be able to swing forward and back and side to side without the grip or position of your hand changing.

> Tip:
>
> It is better initially not to rest your elbow on the arm of the chair, since this inhibits arm movement and makes it more difficult for the pendulum to swing. It may be easier to operate the pendulum standing up, especially at first.

Now you need to train your body to make the pendulum move without any conscious involvement.

Your unconscious is assisting you all the time. That's its purpose. When you're driving, for example, you often move your foot from accelerator to brake and make minor adjustments to your steering without any conscious cognition of what you are doing. It wasn't always like that. When you were learning to drive, every move from pedal to pedal and every turn of the steering wheel was entirely conscious and intentional. After you rehearsed these processes enough times, your body learnt to do it for you.

Most of your everyday behaviour is habitual and unconscious, requiring very little conscious awareness and attention. When you learn any skill it's actually your unconscious body that learns it. Habits are useful for the same reason: your unconscious performs the action without the conscious mind needing to think about it.

You are going to teach your unconscious how to move your arm to move the pendulum – in a similar way to when you taught your unconscious how to drive (or perform some other habitual action if you don't drive).

Fortunately this is simple and your unconscious will learn very quickly.

The two axes of the pendulum

Take a piece of paper and draw a large cross on it, like the one in figure 1.3 – or simply use the diagram as your guide – and then take the steps advised in exercise 1.1. If you have used the pendulum before, but generally do circles rather than axes, then do this exercise so that your body can learn to swing the pendulum along the two axes. Waiting for the pendulum to reverse a circular swing is too time consuming.[2]

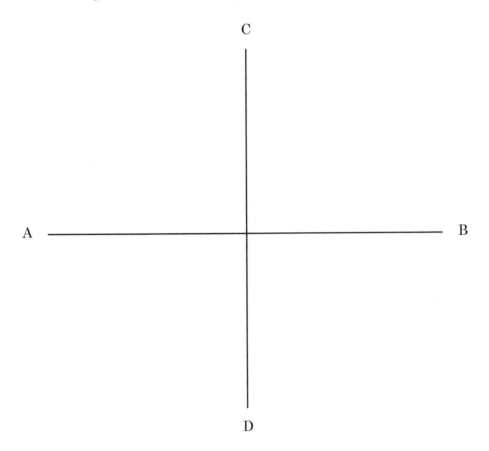

Figure 1.3 The two axes of the pendulum

2   If you have both an axis and a circle as your pendulum responses, that's fine – it's easy for the pendulum to swing from a circle to an axis and vice-versa.

Exercise 1.1: The pendulum swing

1☐ Relax and breathe. Keeping your hand still, let your arm move gently to rock the pendulum from A to B. Let it swing from A to B for a few moments, keeping your eye on the pendulum and the line. Allow it to become automatic. It should move with just a tiny movement of your shoulder. As yet, this movement, though subtle, is still conscious and deliberate.

2☐ Stop the pendulum. Relax and breathe. Gently rock it from C to D. Allow it to become automatic, so it's swinging without trying.

3☐ Repeat this a few times, until it seems to be moving to and fro by itself. Notice that the pendulum is moving without conscious effort.

You can now swing the pendulum along two axes. Well done! The next step is to change the axis of the swing using a transitional circular swing.

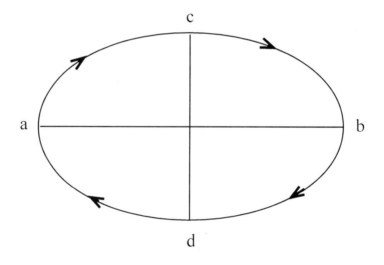

Figure 1.4 Transitional circular swing

Exercise 1.2: Changing the axis

1☐ With the pendulum swinging freely on the A–B axis, encourage it to make a clockwise circular swing. Use figure 1.4 to help orientate the pendulum.

2☐ From the circular swing, encourage the pendulum to settle quickly on the C–D axis.

3⌐ From the C–D axis, encourage the pendulum to move back into the transitional circular swing, and back to the A–B axis.

4⌐ Repeat this a few times, so that it becomes automatic and the pendulum moves effortlessly from axis to axis.

Now that your body knows how to swing the pendulum, you will adopt one axis for YES and another for NO and begin to swing the pendulum without any conscious involvement.

Exercise 1.3: Creating YES and NO axes

1⌐ Say YES to yourself, and notice where in your body you feel the YES. When you have identified its location (in your solar plexus, for example), imagine spreading the feeling up into your shoulder and arm, into your hand and down into the pendulum. Relax and breathe.

2⌐ Keep saying YES to yourself, staying with the feeling and watching the pendulum as it begins to swing. It's important to watch the pendulum since this helps your unconscious to coordinate the subtle movements required. It's okay to give a little conscious encouragement at first, if necessary.

3⌐ Note which axis it decides on (A–B or C–D). Let it swing for a few moments so that your body gets the hang of it. Now stop the pendulum. This is your YES axis.

4⌐ Say No to yourself and feel the No in your body. Identify its location and spread the feeling of the No up to your arm, into your hand and down to the pendulum.

5⌐ Keeping saying No to yourself, and watch the pendulum as it swings along the other axis. Relax and breathe. This is your NO axis.

6⌐ Let the pendulum swing on its NO axis. Now say YES to yourself and focus on the YES. Watch the pendulum change direction and begin to swing on the YES axis – without any conscious effort on your part. The change in swing from one axis to another, whether it's from YES to NO or NO to YES, we shall call a *signal change*.

Well done. Your unconscious has now learnt to move the pendulum for YES and NO, and I'm sure it's very keen to communicate with you! Perhaps the swing is still a bit tentative. That's fine. It will quickly become exuberant! Maybe it already is.

If you have any difficulty, take a break. Then repeat the exercise. Often, when learning something new, just giving yourself a short break from what you're trying to learn means that, when you come back to it, you find you have (that is, your unconscious has) learnt it. Remember to relax and breathe. It's easy. There is no conscious effort involved. You might find it's even better after a night's sleep.

Initial practice

Now that your unconscious can swing the pendulum for you, you can play. You're working in YES/POSITIVE–NO/STRESSED mode (+/– mode). Ask some simple yes-or-no questions of your unconscious. It's very important not to ask anything that is of great significance or stresses your body at this stage. All you're doing now is consolidating the basics of this wonderful new skill. Of course, all your questions need to be answerable by YES or NO. Avoid negative formulations such as I don't like beetroot. It's not at all clear what yes or no would mean in answer to such questions. Be clear and specific in your questions.

> Tip:
>
> Keep focused on your question. If you ask one question and then start thinking of another, the pendulum may start answering the second question that you are in the process of formulating – even though you're expecting an answer to your first question. The pendulum responds to what you are thinking now.

As you do exercise 1.4, give the correct or a false answer inside the square brackets, and observe the pendulum's swing. You will need to give the pendulum a few moments to see whether or not you get a signal change (change of swing from one axis to another).

Exercise 1.4: Initial questions

1□   With your pendulum in hand, relax and breathe. Just taking a breath can often put life into the swing of the pendulum. It's your unconscious body that's moving the pendulum; it can only do this if you're relaxed.

2☐   Say: My name is [. . .]
3☐   Say: My occupation is [. . .]
4☐   Say: My age is [. . .]
5☐   Say: The day today is [. . .]
6☐   Say: I was born in [. . .]
7☐   Say: The weather today is [. . .]

You can get a little more adventurous. Note down the results to exercise 1.5.
Where there are square brackets, insert whatever you like.

Exercise 1.5: More questions

1☐   My favourite holiday activity is [. . .]
2☐   I am getting enough sleep.
3☐   I am happy in my work.
4☐   I drink enough pure water.
5☐   It would benefit me to drink more pure water.
6☐   I am exercising sufficiently.
7☐   It would benefit me to exercise more.
8☐   It would benefit me to exercise more gently.
9☐   It's very relaxing for me to [. . .]
10☐   Right now I feel [. . .]

The questions in exercise 1.5 are not so straightforward because (1) you may
not know the answer; (2) there may be a conflict underlying the response
(for example, you might be happy in your work in certain respects but not
others); (3) there may be stress connected with the issue (if there's a lot of
stress, the pendulum response may be erroneous); (4) the question might
not be explicit enough (for example, I am getting enough sleep is very vague.
Enough sleep for what? To exist? To function? To function optimally? To
function optimally at work, or at home?); (5) the answer you get may not be
what you consciously expect.

If you get a dubious result to a question, check by asking a basic question,
such as My name is [. . .] If you get an erroneous result to this, it means that
one of the questions you've asked has stressed your body. Put the pendulum aside for now. These issues will be addressed later. For now, yes or no
answers to straightforward questions are all we're looking for.

It might be interesting to vary the wording of the questions. The more specific
the question, the more specific and useful the answer will be. You might say:

I am getting enough sleep to perform at the optimum level in my work (which may be very different from getting enough sleep to stay healthy or to perform adequately at work). Or: *My most relaxing holiday activity is [. . .]* The wording of your question is obviously crucial with respect to the response you get. Your intention needs to be very clear.

Indicator change mode

In kinesiology the response of a muscle can have three meanings.

1□ The response of a muscle means either yes or no in answer to a yes-or-no question. The locked muscle represents a YES and the unlocked muscle represents a NO.

2□ The response of a muscle means that the stimulus is stressful or not stressful. A locking muscle indicates the body is not stressed in response to a stimulus; an unlocking muscle indicates the body experiences stress in response to a stimulus. (The stimulus can be a verbal question or statement or can be a physical item introduced into the body's energy field.)

3□ The muscle responds with what is called an indicator change (or, in our terms, signal change). This means that, in response to a stimulus, there is a change in the response of the muscle such that a previously locked muscle now unlocks; or a previously unlocked muscle now locks.

The first two meanings – YES/NO and POSITIVE (unstressed)/STRESSED – you are already familiar with from the discussion in the introduction. With respect to the pendulum, these two types of response happily cohere. We can ask questions and get yes or no answers; we can make statements and get positive or negative responses; and we can introduce stimuli (including verbal and non-verbal statements or challenges) and get a non-stressed or a stressed response. Since these two meanings happily cohere, we'll put them together and call this YES/POSITIVE–NO/STRESSED mode, or +/– mode.

Your patience is requested while I explain the third possible muscle response and additional meaning of a pendulum swing. The muscle responds to a stimulus with what is called an indicator (or signal) change. This means that, in response to a stimulus, there is a change in the response of the muscle, such that a previously locked muscle now unlocks, or a previously unlocked muscle now locks.

The concept of indicator change is very helpful to us for the pendulum because it gives real flexibility. When working in what we will call indicator change mode, or IC mode, instead of swinging to a specific axis for YES and NO, the pendulum will simply change its swing from one axis to the other. In this mode, the pendulum can give a signal change to register either a stress or a benefit, and it doesn't matter which axis it changes to.

It can be time consuming for the pendulum to change its swing, and it can save time if the pendulum only gives a signal change for the option you want. For example, when looking for the resolution to a problem there may be a number of possible remedies. The remedies that produce an indicator change are the ones that will be helpful.

An indicator change, or signal change, means a change of swing from one axis to the other. It doesn't matter whether it has moved from the A–B axis to the C–D axis or vice-versa. Nor does it matter which axis represents YES or NO, since the YES/POSITIVE–NO/STRESSED axes are irrelevant. In indicator change mode, a change of swing from A–B to C–D is an indicator (or signal) change; and a swing from C–D to A–B is an indicator (or signal) change. It's straightforward enough: exercise 1.6 will help you get the hang of it.

Exercise 1.6: IC (indicator change) mode

1⊓ Start with the pendulum swinging on what is normally your YES axis.
2⊓ Now ask for an indicator change. Say: Please give me an indicator change. Watch the pendulum change its swing to the other axis.
3⊓ Ask for an indicator change again, and the pendulum will swing back to the original axis.

It's as simple as that. It's usually a good idea to start the pendulum swinging on the YES/POSITIVE (+) axis, but you will very often be using indicator change mode (IC mode) rather than YES/POSITIVE–NO/STRESSED mode (+/– mode).

How do you activate this mode? Simply through intention. Your body knows what your conscious mind is doing. Have the intention that you are operating in IC mode, and you will be.

This concept is probably the most challenging part of your journey towards expertise in utilizing the therapist within you. If you're beginning to grasp the concept of indicator change mode, everything else will be relatively simple. If you feel you haven't got it yet, that's okay. Read a bit further; it's going to get clearer.

You now have a good idea about:

- ○ What kinesiology is.
- ○ What muscle testing involves.
- ○ How to get a pendulum to work for you.
- ○ The distinction between +/– mode (YES/POSITIVE–NO/STRESSED mode) and IC mode (indicator change mode).

Please maintain your concentration for the next conceptual tool, which you will need in order to use IC mode.

YES–NO director

Imagine you are using +/– mode, and your pendulum is swinging on the YES axis. You ask your body a question. The pendulum continues to swing on the YES/POSITIVE axis. Is the answer yes, or has it stopped working? Change to IC mode and you know instantly whether it's working. Ask the question in IC mode and the pendulum will give a signal change for YES. For the pendulum to maintain its swing on the YES axis (in +/– mode) is not as convincing as when (in IC mode) it changes its swing.

Generally, you'll want an indicator change (a change in the swing of the pendulum) to mean YES/POSITIVE, but it's also possible to make an indicator change mean NO/STRESSED. You can decide whether you want an indicator change to mean YES/POSITIVE or NO/STRESSED by using the YES and NO signals (directors). The YES signal, or director, is activated when your palm (usually the one not holding the pendulum) is open and facing upwards. This is palm mode. The NO signal, or director, is activated when your hand is in the form of a fist and your knuckles are facing upwards. This is knuckles mode.

With your open palm (palm mode) you are asking your pendulum to give you a signal change for YES/TRUE/NO STRESS. In other words, you are asking for an indicator change if the answer is yes or true, or if the stimulus does not produce any stress (YES director).

With your clenched fist (knuckles mode) you are asking your pendulum to give you a signal change for NO/FALSE/STRESS. In other words, you will get an indicator change if the answer is no or false, or if the stimulus produces stress (NO director).

The explanation is a bit wordy, but the principle is simple enough. If that's not clear, just take a moment to read through this explanation again. Take a break first . . .

Well done! The examples that follow demonstrate the use of YES–NO director. Keep in mind that with the palm mode there will be an indicator change if the statement is true or the answer is yes; with the knuckles mode there will be an indicator change if the statement is false or the answer is no. After looking at the examples, do exercise 1.7

Examples:

1   *I am a human being* [palm mode]. There is (fortunately) an indicator change, meaning *yes*.

2   *I am a man* [knuckles mode]. Fortunately for me, no indicator change. The statement is *true*. There would only have been an indicator change if the statement had been false.

3   *I was born in the UK* [palm mode]. There is no indicator change. This means this is *not* the case.

4   *I was born in the UK* [knuckles mode]. There is an indicator change, meaning *no* or *false*. This means I was not born in the UK.

5   *I was born in east Africa* [palm mode]. There is an indicator change. The statement is correct.

When using IC mode the default will be an indicator change for YES/TRUE/ NO STRESS. When you are practised in using YES–NO director you won't need to put your hand out when you are using the default; that is, when you are asking for an indicator change for YES/TRUE/NO STRESS. All you will need is your intention.

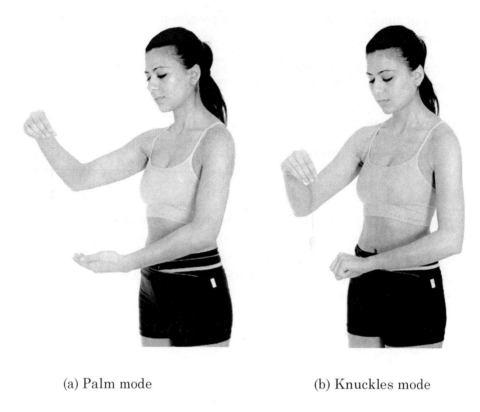

(a) Palm mode   (b) Knuckles mode

Figure 1.5 YES–NO director (palm mode & knuckles mode)

Normally you will want an indicator change for YES (palm mode). However, there are times when you may have a list of questions and expect a positive answer to most of them. It may then be easier to use knuckles mode and have the indicator change for NO. Or you may simply want confirmation that the answer really is NO. If you want an indicator change for NO/FALSE/ STRESS, use knuckles mode. Once you're very familiar with the YES–NO director, even for knuckles mode you can use your intention rather than actually clenching your fist – do this simply by imagining using the mode. But, for now, physically use the mode since it helps to clarify your intention.

Exercise 1.7: Using YES–NO director (palm & knuckles modes)

1□   Have the pendulum swinging on your YES axis, and have the intention of using IC mode.

2⌐ Say *My name is [YOUR NAME]* and apply palm mode. [Pendulum shows an indicator change (expressing yes).]

3⌐ Say *My name is [FALSE NAME]* and apply palm mode. [Pendulum shows no indicator change.]

4⌐ Say *My name is [FALSE NAME]* and apply the knuckles mode. [Pendulum shows an indicator change (expressing no, that's not your name).]

When you are comfortable working with IC mode and +/– mode, you can decide which you want to use at any time, rather than necessarily using the modes suggested in the text. The important thing is to be clear in your own mind whether you are looking for a signal change for YES or a signal change for NO.

2
Preparations & Precautions

Like many other people, when I learnt to use the pendulum I was very excited and began to ask lots of interesting and significant questions about my childhood, and about other people's actions and motivations – aware that my unconscious doesn't miss a trick, understands far more than my conscious mind, and is the repertory of all my experience.

But very soon I frequently began to get nonsensical and anomalous answers in response to my questioning. It often seemed that the more meaningful the question, the more meaningless the answer. And so, like many others, I abandoned the pendulum, disillusioned – until I discovered kinesiology.

This chapter is about applying kinesiology principles to ensure that the pendulum provides accurate responses. Generally speaking, the unconscious is meant to be just that – unconscious. It wants to help us, but isn't necessarily going to reveal all its secrets. There's a good reason, I think, why we can't generally hold on to our dreams. We're not meant to remember them. They are (usually) intended for unconscious use only. The unconscious isn't anyway like a memory storage system. We live in the present. It's only unprocessed traumas that are stuck in the body that we need to resolve (more of this later). The body will help us to resolve these issues. It's not a playground.

Life tracks

From conception, our experience is registered and recorded in the unconscious body. This is a Freudian notion verified in clinical practice.

That the unconscious body has access to all experience doesn't mean, how-ever, that this knowledge can be freely summoned up by the conscious mind. Freud likened the unconscious to the child's toy, the mystic writing pad. The child writes or draws on the mystic writing pad with a sharp instrument and what is written appears clearly on the surface of this pad. When the child gets tired of these scribbles, he or she lifts up the plastic surface of the pad and the surface once again becomes clear. The child can start all over again with a clean slate.

The surface of the pad Freud compares to the conscious mind. The conscious mind is limited in what it can hold at one time (seven chunks of information – plus or minus two – is all the conscious mind can manage at a given mo-ment); and memory (that which can be consciously recalled – equivalent to Freud's notion of the *preconscious*) is selective and often vague, fragmentary and faulty.

But if you lift up the plastic sheet and look underneath, you can see im-printed there the traces of everything that was ever scribbled on the sheet. This is like the unconscious: all experiences, including those in the womb, are imprinted in the unconscious. Nothing is lost. Everything is indelibly recorded. Much, including (for most people) most pre-verbal experiences, can never be made conscious; but the tracks are nonetheless there and the body can communicate about them through the pendulum.

This is borne out in clinical practice. Very frequently, as they travel to the source trauma, clients return not only to their early childhood years but even to birth and their life in the womb itself. The body 'remembers' what hap-pened before birth. Of course no one can recall the content of conversations from the womb, but the body does know, for example, when the mother was depressed, suffered some trauma, or if he or she was unwanted.

We know this intuitively: every experience, including those about which we have no conscious memory, influences us. We learn through experience. How else could you be affected by things that happened before any conscious recol-lection unless there is such an impression of it in the body?

The impression of all experience inheres in the body and, where the im-pression is traumatic, it will continue to affect your life whenever your current life experience connects with it in any way. It's like a groove that, as life revolves, you continually fall back in to. Fortunately, with the right methods, any trauma can be resolved (although for some the assistance of a good therapist may be helpful).

Respecting your unconscious

The unconscious body carries the impressions of all experience. Your body knows everything that's happened to you. Why then does the pendulum sometimes give erroneous and completely nonsensical responses?

Not all unconscious information is able to be readily communicated. Remember that your body systems function in a completely different way from the conscious mind and realm of thought. In addition, your unconscious knows much better than your conscious mind what is good for you. If you ask questions of your unconscious that it believes it is not safe for the conscious mind to access, it won't give you reliable answers. It's as simple as that. This is true of the pendulum; it is equally true of hypnosis. If a part of your experience has been blotted out of conscious recollection, it is for very good reason. Hypnosis won't necessarily suddenly reveal those experiences; nor will the pendulum.

There are ways of getting there, of course. You can work with the wisdom of the unconscious – the therapist within you – to make those experiences safe. Then the unconscious may well make them available to conscious recall. It is not uncommon for survivors of abuse, for example, to have lost periods of their past where perhaps months or even years are difficult to recall in any detail. This is a self-protection mechanism. But as the traumas associated with the abusive experiences are addressed in therapy, it gradually becomes safe for the memories to emerge.

This brings us to a fundamental law. The first law of the pendulum: always ask permission for whatever work you do with the pendulum. This is worth restating.

Caution:

Always ask permission for work you do with the pendulum.

If you suspect there is anything that might be controversial about what you want to ask of your unconscious, then ask permission before you ask your questions. If permission is not granted, leave it alone. It is important to trust and respect your unconscious. If you persist in asking when you have not been given permission, you will get phoney answers. It is also disrespectful to your unconscious. Respecting your unconscious, which of course is respecting yourself, is very important. It can be helpful to see your unconscious as an entity separate from your conscious mind – which of course it is. Your conscious mind didn't create you and doesn't maintain you. Your unconscious body, which is an integral part of nature, a creation of the universe, gives you life and substance. You have a duty to take care of it. Indeed, taking care of yourself is your first responsibility.

If you are denied permission to work on something, find out what you can work with. As you resolve these issues, gradually, you will gain access to those things that were initially denied conscious access.

The pendulum's truth

If you follow the guidelines given in this book, the pendulum will give you highly reliable and accurate information to help you regain and maintain the health of your whole being. It may or may not tell you God's Truth. That is to say, it will give you the truth of your unconscious body's perceptions and interpretations. These should not be confused with objective reality (whatever that would be – should such a thing exist). The version of your unconscious body may not accord with anyone else's version of reality – especially regarding childhood events.

Often in therapy a client will not remember details of their life which they assume to have been traumatic and ask for my help to remember them. I acknowledge that the facts of what happened may be of great importance to them. But I let them know that I have no privileged access to their past. I explain that my task is to help them heal, and if this leads to clearer and more detailed recall of past events, that's to be welcomed; but I can't know whether the events we uncover occurred precisely as is recalled or not. What matters is healing, not establishing facts.

My attitude to the revelations of the pendulum is the same. I don't know whether the information uncovered accords with the historical facts. It may well be that it does, but I don't know. I know that, used properly and carefully, the pendulum gives us access to the amazing wisdom of the unconscious body and provides a wonderful healing tool. But it should not be regarded as an infallible historian or prophet. For this reason, I advise against using the pendulum to learn the truth about some detail in your past. It certainly won't stand up in court.

The techniques and exercises in the next few pages ensure that your body is functioning properly for accurate pendulum work. If your body requires them, the corrections will also be particularly beneficial in themselves.

Stress and the central meridian

If an issue that you are addressing is particularly stressful, the pendulum may give anomalous results. Under stress the central meridian,[1] which acts as a reservoir of energy and is also the meridian associated with the brain, can become over-energized.

> **Caution:**
>
> Stress can create over-energy in the central meridian and lead to false results.

When the central meridian is over-energized, the pendulum may give the opposite results to those it should give. It is not that the unconscious doesn't want to give you the correct answer (since you have been given permission), but that the stress of the issue has overwhelmed you, over-energizing the central meridian and leading to false readings. Fortunately, there is a straightforward remedy.

Pre-test # 1
Central meridian over-energy: TEST

1☐   Have the pendulum swinging on your YES axis. You are using +/– mode.

2☐   Using two fingers on your free hand, deliberately sweep up the centre of your body from your groin to just below the middle of your bottom lip, along the path of the central meridian (see figure 2.1, which also shows the path of the governing meridian), as if doing up a zip ('zipping up'). Your fingers can be in contact with your body or up to two inches off it.

---

1   Often also called the Central Vessel (CV), this energy channel runs from the groin to just below the middle of your bottom lip.

3☐   Notice the pendulum swing. (But be careful that the action of trac-
     ing your central meridian has not unduly disturbed the motion of the
     pendulum.) All being well, the swing should continue as before on the
     YES axis. (If the swing changes from the YES/POSITIVE axis to the
     NO/STRESSED axis, there is central meridian over-energy.)
4☐   Now sweep in the opposite direction, down the centre of your body
     from just below your bottom lip to groin, as if undoing a zip ('zipping
     down'). If all is well, the pendulum should change its swing from the
     YES/POSITIVE axis to the NO/STRESSED axis. (If it doesn't, it prob-
     ably indicates central meridian over-energy.)
5☐   If you have had contrary results in (3) and (4), do the correction.

This is what's going on. The energies of the body flow continuously in one
direction around the body in channels called meridians. Tracing along the
path of the meridian in the direction of the energy flow is normally enjoyed
by the body, since it encourages the flow of energy (qi) in and through the
meridian, benefiting the organ–gland system it serves. The pendulum indicates this with a YES/POSITIVE response.

However, if the meridian is blocked and has too much qi (and so is over-
energized) the last thing it wants is more energy. Tracing the meridian in
the direction of the energy flow (upwards, in the case of the central meridian)
is only encouraging a greater concentration of qi in that meridian, which is
already over-energized. The pendulum registers a stress to the body. On the
other hand, tracing a blocked and over-energized meridian backwards is a
relief to the body, since the flow of energy into that meridian is being discouraged. The pendulum registers a positive response.

To ensure that the pendulum does not give false results, correct over-energy
immediately.

You can also check the governing meridian for over-energy. You may need to
do the first half of the meridian trace with one hand, then take over with the
other to complete the path.

Central meridian over-energy corrections

There are two options. Either will resolve the over-energy. While the meridian flush can be done in 30 seconds or so, the harmonizing posture takes a

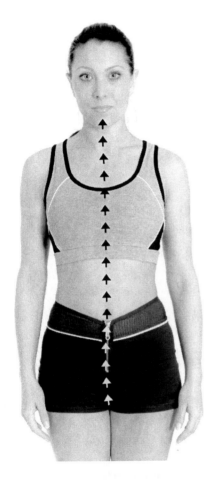
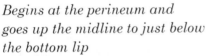
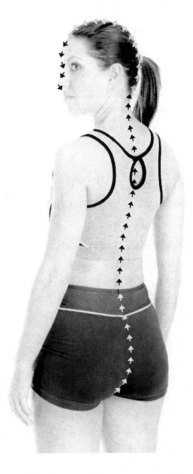

Begins at the perineum and goes up the midline to just below the bottom lip

Begins at the coccyx and and goes up the midline, over the head, to just below the nose

(a) Central meridian

(b) Governing meridian

Figure 2.1 The paths of the central and governing meridians

few minutes, but leaves you feeling wonderful. The harmonizing posture is also excellent for correcting hyperstress (a significant condition when the body is in a state of self-protection and less amenable to therapy – see below), and leaves you feeling centred and calm. Do the harmonizing posture any time you're feeling overwhelmed.

PRE-TEST # 1
Central meridian flush: CORRECTION (1)

Run your two fingers up and down the length of the meridian a number of times. End with two or three deliberate upward strokes. Remember to relax and breathe. (A good breath helps to keep that pendulum swinging!)

PRE-TEST # 1
Harmonizing posture: CORRECTION (2)

1☐   Stretch your arms out in front of you with the backs of your hands touching each other.
2☐   Put your right hand over your left and interlock your fingers, with your arms crossed at the wrists.
3☐   Bring your interlocked hands under and up, resting them on your chest.
4☐   With your legs straight, put your left foot over your right, so that your legs are crossed at the ankles.
5☐   Breathe through your nose, putting your tongue to the top of your mouth just behind your top teeth.
6☐   Breathe out through your mouth, putting your tongue to the floor of your mouth.
7☐   Continue breathing in through your nose and out through your mouth in this manner.
8☐   Bring to mind an image of nature's harmony (such as a pink rose).
9☐   Maintain your posture and your breathing as you relax and focus on this image for a few minutes.

Repeat the test for central meridian reversal. Now that the imbalance has been corrected, tracing the meridian upwards and downwards will give the appropriate responses.

If central meridian reversal begins to happen frequently with a particular issue, or persists even after the corrections, you may need to defuse the stress before you can do anything else. Very gently place your hand on your forehead for several minutes while focusing on the issue. This is a brilliant method to defuse stress, which we'll explore in detail later.[2]

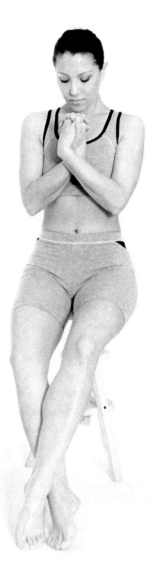

Tips:

If ever your pendulum results seem strange or you suspect them to be inaccurate, check for central meridian over-energy, and of course check you have permission to proceed.

When dealing with a particularly stressful issue, after the pendulum responds to your question check for central meridian reversal.

Figure 2.2
The harmonizing posture

---

2   It occasionally happens that, in relation to a particular issue, the central meridian will keep registering over-energy, despite all your efforts. If this happens, the issue is too stressful to deal with directly on this occasion. You may need to try a different approach, such as starting with a less stressful manifestation of the issue, or you may need to come back to the issue again when you are feeling more resourceful.

Hydration

The human body is composed of 70–80 per cent water. The brain has an even higher proportion of water – or ought to. The body's electrical system is unable to operate reliably if it is dehydrated. The majority of people are dehydrated – many severely. According to one authority, many chronic diseases are a result of chronic dehydration.[3] Probably the simplest action you can take to improve your health dramatically is to drink pure water. Most of us should be drinking at least two litres a day. When ill or stressed or in hot weather it is even more.

Other fluids are no substitute for water. Fruit juices and other drinks aren't recognized as water by the body. When you drink water your body recognizes that you are ingesting water and can immediately release reserve supplies. Other drinks have first to be digested. Tea, coffee and alcoholic drinks are diuretics and dehydrate you by flushing out the water in your body. Carbonated (fizzy) drinks are also dehydrating.

It can take a little while to get used to drinking pure water. There's no obligation to start drinking two litres a day immediately. Gradually increase your water intake.

At the beginning of every pendulum session it is necessary to test for hydration (pre-test # 2). Dehydration is not only detrimental to health but, since the proper functioning of the body's electrical circuits depends on water, proper hydration is another requirement for accurate pendulum work. If you are dehydrated the electrical signals in your body may not be properly transmitted and your results may be erroneous.

PRE-TEST # 2
Hydration: TEST

1☐ Have the pendulum swinging freely on the YES axis.
2☐ Say: *Water*.
3☐ If the pendulum swings to NO/STRESSED you need to make the correction.

---

3 Dr F. Batmanghelidj, *Your Body's Many Cries For Water* (Tagman Press, 2000).

The correction is singularly unsurprising.

PRE-TEST # 2
Hydration: CORRECTION

1⸆   Drink some water. Sip – don't gulp.

2⸆   With the pendulum swinging on the YES axis, check you've drunk enough water by saying again: *Water.*

3⸆   If there is no signal change you are sufficiently hydrated to continue.

You can use the pendulum to find out how much water you should be drinking (exercise 2.1).

Exercise 2.1: General hydration

1⸆   Check for central meridian over-energy. Correct if necessary.

2⸆   Use indicator change mode (IC mode). Ask: *Should I be drinking at least one glass of water a day?*[4] (Use YES director: palm mode.)

3⸆   The response is almost certainly YES (indicator change).

4⸆   Ask: *At least two glasses?*

5⸆   The response again will be YES (indicator change).

6⸆   Ask: *At least three glasses?*

7⸆   Keep going until there is no indicator change. If there is no indicator change on At least eight glasses, for example, it means you need at least seven glasses of water per day.

Remember that any response you get from the pendulum derives from all the information your unconscious body processes today. You can ask about the future (exercise 2.2), but the assessment is based on today's conditions. Compare it to a weather forecast. Accurate predictions may be given for the next 72 hours or so (I'm just guessing); beyond that (or whatever the figure is), predictions becomes less reliable. Weather predictions beyond the next

---

4   Use whatever measure makes sense to you (pints, litres or whatever). If you use the measure of glasses, be clear in your own mind the size of the glass you're referring to.

week (again, just guessing) may be based more on the weather of previous years than measurable activity today and are not necessarily reliable. You can find out the opinion of your unconscious body today, but remember to ask again as soon as appropriate or applicable (you can ask the pendulum when to check again); the response may be very different.

Exercise 2.2: Hydration for the future

1☐   Say: *I should drink x glasses of water for at least the next one day.*
2☐   The response will almost certainly be YES.
3☐   Say: *At least two days.*
4☐   In all probability the answer is YES.
5☐   Continue until no indicator change (if using IC mode). For example, if there is no indicator change when you say *At least five days*, then you need to drink x glasses for at least four days. After four days, check again.

You might need to consider weeks rather than days. Say: *Should I measure in weeks?* If so: say: *At least the next week?* If yes: *At least the next two weeks?* And so on. After this period has elapsed, check again to see if the number is different.

> **Tip:**
>
> You can adapt the procedure in exercise 2.1 whenever you want the pendulum to provide a measure of quantity; and you can adapt the procedure in exercise 2.2 whenever you want a measure of time.

Do you want to find out whether your body prefers still bottled mineral water or filtered tap water? You can ask (exercise 2.3). It's possible that the results might be different with different brands of mineral water, according to the material of the container (glass or plastic), with tap water from different areas of the country, or depending on the filter. It might be helpful to have the mineral water and tap water in front of you and to take a little drink of each – but this isn't strictly necessary if your body is familiar with them both already.

Exercise 2.3: Water preference

1☐   Using indicator change mode (IC mode) and palm mode (YES director), ask: *Does my body have a preference for either mineral or (filtered) tap water?* (An indicator change would mean the answer is YES.)[5]

2☐   Ask: *Does my body prefer (filtered) tap water?* (No indicator change would mean the answer is NO.)

3☐   Ask: *Does my body prefer still mineral water?* (An indicator change would mean the answer is YES.)

Switching

If the body's electrical circuits are not functioning correctly the brain can confuse left and right, up and down, and forwards and backwards, leading to errors in thinking and processing. Problems here can again lead to erroneous results. Checking all three circuits for possible switching, and correcting as necessary, is another preliminary consideration.

Before learning how to test for and correct switching, you need to appreciate the principle of polarity.

Different areas of the body have different polarities. Each finger has a specific polarity. Thumbs are neutral. To ensure that electro-magnetic polarities do not interfere with our tests and corrections, always use a neutral touch unless there is a specific reason not to. Adjoining fingers have opposite polarities, so if you use two adjoining fingers from the same hand you have a positive and a negative polarity, which creates a neutral touch.

Caution:

Unless otherwise specified, always use a neutral touch: either all four fingers, two adjoining fingers, or the thumb.

---

5   I'd be very surprised if your body was happy with drinking adequate quantities of tap water. In my experience testing students and clients, drinking a lot of tap water usually creates severe stress to the body.

Left–right switching

Checking for left–right switching (pre-test # 3) is necessary to ensure accurate results with the pendulum. It may also be helpful for people with dyslexia who confuse left and right and the letters *b* and *d*, for example. The correction appears to unblock neurological pathways in the brain, including the corpus callosum which links the two brain hemispheres.

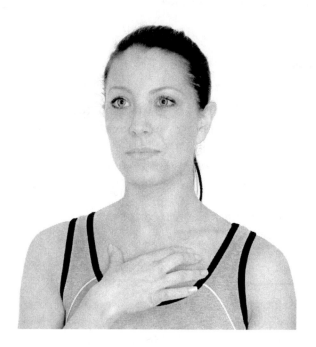

Figure 2.3 The ends of the kidney meridian (K27s)

PRE-TEST # 3
Left–right switching: TEST

1☐   To check for this, with the pendulum swinging on the YES/POSITIVE axis, use the thumb and two fingers of your free hand (for a neutral touch) and firmly (i.e. with moderate pressure) hold the ends of your kidney meridian, bilaterally – that is, on both sides of the body (figure 2.3). (The kidney meridian starts underneath the foot and ends at the top of the chest just underneath the clavicle and to the side of the sternum. The end of the kidney meridian is a very important point in kinesiology and traditional Chinese medicine. It's called the K27: the 27th acupoint on the kidney meridian.)

2☐   If there are no problems, as you hold the K27s the pendulum will continue to swing on the YES/POSITIVE axis.

3☐   If the pendulum changes its swing to the NO/STRESSED axis, the correction is necessary.

PRE-TEST # 3
Left–right switching: CORRECTION

Put down the pendulum: you need both hands.

1☐   Put the palm of one hand flat over the navel and hold it there.

2☐   With the other hand, again using a neutral touch, massage the K27 points for about 15 or 20 seconds.

3☐   Swap the positions of the hands and repeat, remembering to breathe.

4☐   If you once again get a change to NO/STRESSED, repeat the correction.

Now you can test for left–right switching again. This time when you touch the K27 points the pendulum should maintain the same direction of its swing, indicating that there is no longer a problem. If there is again a signal change, you didn't do the correction for long enough. Repeat it.

Up–down switching

Test for up–down switching (pre-test # 4). When up–down switching occurs, the brain seems to confuse messages from the upper body with messages from the lower body and vice-versa. The correction seems to integrate the functionings of the cerebral cortex (the thinking area of the brain) with the deeper and more primitive limbic areas of the brain associated with feeling. Correcting up–down switching not only ensures that the body's electrical system is working properly but can help people who are too much in their head and can't seem to get in touch with their feelings and, conversely, those who can't seem to get out of their feelings and use their head.

The correction procedure is similar to that of left–right switching. The points to check are at the end of the central meridian (which you are now familiar with: it runs up the front of the body from the perineum to just below the middle of your bottom lip) and at the end of the governing meridian (which runs along the back of the body from the coccyx, up the spine, over the centre of the head and down to just underneath the nose).

PRE-TEST # 4
Up–down switching: TEST

1☐   With the pendulum swinging on the YES/POSITIVE axis, with two fingers and the thumb of your free hand (for a neutral touch), touch just below your bottom lip and beneath the nose simultaneously.
2☐   If the pendulum changes its swing to NO/STRESSED do the correction.

PRE-TEST # 4
Up–down switching: CORRECTION

1☐   Place one hand over the navel and hold it there.
2☐   With the other, using a neutral touch, massage beneath the nose and just below your bottom lip.
3☐   Swap hands and repeat.

Repeat the test. The pendulum should retain its swing on the YES/POSITIVE axis. If you again get a change to NO/STRESSED, repeat the correction.

Forward–backward switching

Test for forward–backward switching (pre-test # 5). If there is switching here the body will confuse messages from the front and back of the body. The front of the brain relates to associational thinking and the back of the brain is where memories are stored, and also where sensory information is processed. If the pathways between the front and back of your brain become blocked, thinking can become divorced from past experiences and you run the risk either of not learning from the past, or of being too preoccupied with the past.

PRE-TEST # 5
Forward–backward switching: TEST

1☐   With your free hand, neutral touch the tip of the coccyx. Be careful that the movement itself does not disturb the swing of the pendulum.
2☐   If there is an indicator change, go to the correction.

PRE-TEST # 5
Forward–backward switching: CORRECTION

1☐   Place one hand over the navel.
2☐   With the other hand, using a neutral touch, massage the tip of the coccyx.
3☐   Swap hands and repeat.

Retest. There should be no change from YES/POSITIVE to NO/STRESSED. If there is, repeat the correction.

Tip:

When using the pendulum has become familiar, it's usually possible to feel the pendulum as it begins to change its swing. You may want to take this as evidence of an indicator change without waiting for the swing to change axis completely. This is usually perfectly okay, but be cautious. Sometimes the indicator may swing to the other axis, and then swing back to the original axis. When this happens, it does not signify an indicator change. Perhaps it's just the unconscious reconsidering its response or making some adjustment.

Balanced ionization

There's one more test you need to carry out to ensure the body's electrical systems are working properly (pre-test # 6). This test is to ensure you have a balance of positive and negative ions.

Many electrical devices in the environment, including computers and fluorescent lighting, give out positive ions. Negative ions come from vegetation and rain, for example. Imbalances in your environment can affect your body's electro-magnetic circuits and change the polarities of your body.[6] Stress can also affect your breathing and disrupt your ionization balance. It is imperative that the electro-magnetic polarities of your body are correct when you touch parts of your body during the kinesiology therapy.

Inhaling through the right nostril promotes positive ions and stimulates left-hemisphere dominance; inhaling through the left nostril promotes negative ions and stimulates right-hemisphere dominance. As we breathe, every 90 minutes or so the emphasis of our breathing changes from one nostril to the other, affecting the ionization balance.

PRE-TEST # 6
Balanced ionization: TEST

1☐   Let the pendulum swing on the YES/POSITIVE axis and, with your free hand, use a neutral touch (thumb or two fingers) to block the left nostril. Breathe calmly and deeply in and out through the right nostril. A signal change signifies a problem.

2☐   Ensure the pendulum is swinging on the YES/POSITIVE axis. Now block the right nostril with a neutral touch. Breathe calmly and deeply in and out of the left nostril. A signal change signifies a problem.

If there is an indicator change breathing through either nostril, do the correction.

---

6   Don't attempt to use the pendulum under fluorescent lighting or close to computers. It may well affect the accuracy of your results.

PRE-TEST # 6
Balanced ionization: CORRECTION

1☐ With one hand let the pendulum swing freely on one axis. For this it's easier to use the IC mode with the YES director (palm mode). Put the tongue to the roof of the mouth, just behind the front teeth and hold it there throughout the correction.

2☐ Block the left nostril and breathe in deeply through the right nostril to the count of four.

3☐ Block the right nostril and breathe out through the left nostril to the count of eight.

4☐ Still blocking the right nostril, breathe in through the left nostril to the count of four.

5☐ Block the left nostril and breathe out to the count of eight.

6☐ Still blocking the left nostril, breathe in through the right, and so on.

7☐ Continue until there is an indicator change, which shows that the problem has been rectified.

Hyperstress

Hyperstress is identified in kinesiology when a muscle is unable to turn off. This is a problem in kinesiology because, unless tested for, a hyperstressed condition will be mistaken for an unstressed condition, since a locked muscle is usually taken to signify absence of stress.

There is no evidence I'm aware of to suggest that hyperstress adversely affects the movement of the pendulum; however, the hyperstressed state is highly undesirable in itself, and corrections are less likely to be effective since the body is on guard and in a self-protective state. Check for hyperstress as one of your initial tests.

PRE-TEST # 7
Hyperstress: TEST

1☐ Using IC mode (and palm mode), make this statement: My body is receptive and amenable to change.

2☐   If you get a signal change, you're fine. If you don't, your body is in hyperstress. (When my body is in hyperstress I still get a pendulum response but, instead of swinging to the opposite axis to give a positive response, the pendulum makes erratic circles. The response your body gives might be different to this.) Do the correction.

PRE-TEST # 7
Hyperstress: CORRECTION

1☐   Still holding the pendulum in one hand, place your other hand over you forehead very gently, touching your frontal eminences (the two bumps that appear prominent in some people between the eyebrows and the hairline), but without applying any pressure (also see figure 5.1).

2☐   Hold until you get a signal change (suggesting the hyperstress is corrected).

3☐   Repeat the test. If you still don't get a signal change when you make the statement, repeat the correction.

Tip:

If your pendulum does not swing entirely to the other axis to give a standard reading it is not giving a definitive YES/POSITIVE or NO/STRESSED answer. However, a swing that's three-quarters of the way there, for example, may be giving you a helpful message – that you're three-quarters of the way there.

The conscious sway

You are now very nearly ready to use the pendulum with an assurance of its accuracy. There is one final thing to learn.

You saw earlier how easy it is to influence the pendulum through the desire and wishes of your conscious mind. Take a moment to experience this now (exercise 2.4).

Exercise 2.4: Conscious override

1☐   Using +/– mode, have your pendulum swinging on the YES axis.
2☐   Say to yourself, My name is [YOUR NAME]. The pendulum maintains its swing on the YES axis.
3☐   Say: My name is [SOME OTHER NAME]. The pendulum now swings to the NO axis. This much is familiar and the expected response.
4☐   Now say: My name is [NOT YOUR NAME]. Yes. Yes. Yes. Watch the pendulum swing to the YES axis, influenced by your repetition of 'yes', even though it's not your name.
5☐   With the pendulum now swinging on the YES axis, say: My name is [YOUR NAME]. No. No. No. Watch the pendulum swing to NO, influenced by your repetition of 'no', even though it is your name.[7]

This demonstrates how easy it is for the pendulum to be influenced by what you want. You don't have to be saying yes out loud to get a YES result; just wishing it strongly would be enough. This is why pendulum aficionados often advocate a mind-clearing exercise as part of the preparations, and emphasize how important it is to keep your mind clear and have no expectations.

There is a quicker way. It is not necessarily infallible, and of course it is good to keep the mind clear and have no expectations, but the pendulum mode seems to be very effective in overriding conscious wishes and desires. Without the pendulum mode you might not know for sure whether the pendulum is simply telling you what you want to hear.

Kinesiologists use a number of finger (or hand) modes to ask questions of the body non-verbally. You are already familiar with the YES–NO director which, although presented for the first time in this text, is based on the same principles. You will encounter more finger modes later. How they work I'm afraid I'm completely at a loss to say. Perhaps it's just a convention to clarify our intentions. The sceptical mind might insist that this is the only explanation. But there does seem to be more to it.

---

7 If the pendulum maintains its truthful swing, it may be that you have a particularly strong moral code prohibiting falsehood and lying. This was the experience of an Irish kinesiologist with a Roman Catholic background who did this exercise. I doubt Anglo-Saxons with a Protestant background, like myself, have such scruples. Let me know if I'm wrong.

One renowned kinesiologist, Bruce Dewe MD, reports that, in response to his request, people from different parts of the world sent in their finger-mode discoveries. The amazing outcome, I'm reliably informed, was that the finger modes sent in by different people from various parts of the world tallied with each other – despite being discovered entirely independently. In other words, apparently, different people independently came up with the same finger mode for the same thing.

On the other hand, different branches of kinesiology use the same finger mode for different purposes, perhaps suggesting that the intention of the user is the most important factor. I've heard one kinesiologist who came up with a couple of interesting finger modes claim that, while other modes are really just about intention, his finger modes are more than that![8] (I would make the same claim for my modes.) It has been suggested that the mudras of Hinduism and Buddhism have an equivalence with finger modes.

The pendulum mode

The pendulum mode is a discovery I made – or, rather, that my unconscious revealed to me – some time before I realized what it could do. But the pendulum mode is crucial to the accurate application of the pendulum. Without it, this book would probably not have been written. This is what it does: the pendulum mode helps to prevent conscious wishes from overriding the message from the unconscious body.

The finger position is not easy to describe in words, so please also refer to figure 2.4. The mode involves the middle finger and the thumb. (It makes no difference which hand you use for any of the finger modes). First identify the points on the finger and thumb which will make contact.

1▢   Look at the back of your hand. The thumb point is halfway between the bottom of the nail and the upper thumb joint. But the point is not on the back of the thumb but rather on the side of the thumb that you can see when looking at the back of your hand.
2▢   Now look again at the back of your hand. The middle finger point is level with the bottom of the fingernail, but not on the back of the finger but rather on the side closest to the little finger.

8   This was the late Alan Sales, who made a significant contribution to energy kinesiology.

3⌐   Simply move your middle finger across your thumb to connect those
      two points. This is the pendulum mode.

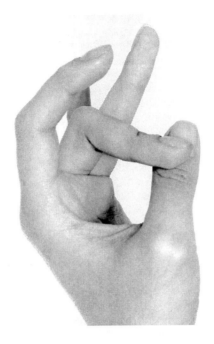

Figure 2.4 The pendulum mode

Do the conscious override exercise again. This time, apply the pendulum
mode with your free hand. You should notice that even though you say,

> *My name is* [YOUR TRUE NAME]. *No. No. No.*

the pendulum now swings to (or maintains) the YES axis. And when you
say,

> *My name is* [FALSE NAME]. *Yes. Yes. Yes.*

the pendulum now swings to (or maintains) the NO axis.

It is not necessary to use the pendulum mode all the time – just double check
using the mode if you suspect that the answer the pendulum has given you
may be more in accordance with your desires than the truth.

I find I rarely need to use the pendulum mode any more. Just knowing that I can and will use it if I suspect my desires are getting the upper hand has a constraining influence in itself. I suggest you use it frequently at first, and then whenever you think your wishes may be overriding the truth.

In chapter 4 you will begin to learn some of kinesiology's particularly powerful corrections. But first, here's how to use the pendulum to help someone else.

3
The Surrogate Pendulum

Rather than teaching someone else to use the pendulum, and the methods described here, you can be a surrogate for the pendulum to express the unconscious communications of someone else.

In kinesiology a surrogate is often used when the person receiving the treatment is infirm, paralysed or too young to be muscle tested. If you have young children, you can use the pendulum to find out what the problem is and how you can help – exactly as you would use it with your own issues. You can be a surrogate for anyone. It's quicker than teaching them how to use the pendulum.

All you need is their permission and physical contact with the person you're surrogating for. Ideally, hold that person's hand. The palm of the hand (or sole of the foot) is the most reliable conductor of energy for this purpose; but it's usually okay to be touching any part of that person, even over clothing.[1]

When working with another person it is vital to ask permission – not only of the person's conscious mind, but also of their unconscious body (using the pendulum). If you are working with young children, ask for permission of their unconscious body through the pendulum. With permission granted, all

---

1 Many kinesiologists work with people over the telephone, where there is no direct contact, muscle testing themselves as a surrogate. This involves something of a leap of faith. However, even without invoking psychic powers (or belief in the union of everything in the universe) it can be readily acknowledged that a great deal of information is transmitted through the voice which is read unconsciously. For therapists who muscle test themselves in the presence of the client but without physical contact, additional information is available from the visible physiology of the client. It's also possible that we read the energy of a situation (in the same way as we pick up an atmosphere). However, surrogacy using direct contact with the person produces demonstrably reliable results.

the pre-tests should be done. For a summary of the pre-tests, go to the beginning of the next chapter.

When possible, it is most effective to perform the test and the correction on the person you are surrogating for (rather than on yourself); use the pendulum solely for the other person's unconscious communication. For example, zip up their central meridian, or massage their K27s, rather than your own.

If for some reason the test or correction cannot be performed on the other person, you can do it on yourself. This can still be very effective, but you must remain in physical contact with the other person while the test and correction are carried out. It's fine to break physical contact between questions, but contact must be maintained while requesting a response from the pendulum and while performing the correction (if done on the surrogate).

Tip:

While working as a surrogate, it's vital that both you and the person you're surrogating for are focused on what you're doing. If you or the other person's mind begins to wonder, the pendulum will stop working accurately.

How surrogacy works

This kind of surrogacy seems contrary to received wisdom and common sense and is based on the energy model. If you are sceptical, I don't blame you; just try it!

When you are in physical contact with another person, your energy fields are united. This means that your body can respond to the information in the unconscious body of the other person, and your arm or shoulder will move the pendulum in accordance with their unconscious communications. Your intention to act as a surrogate means that the pendulum responds to the other's unconscious rather than your own.

Kinesiologists use this energy-field connection all the time when working with clients. For example, the client's body, during a muscle test, is able to choose a remedy that he or she has no notion of. This is possible because the energetic connection of client and therapist (and the therapist's knowledge of the remedy) means that the client's body can indicate which remedy is most beneficial.

Being a surrogate

To test another using yourself as a surrogate:

1☐ Do the pre-tests and corrections on yourself.
2☐ Use the pendulum to do the pre-tests on the other person. Correct as necessary.
3☐ Use the pendulum to ask their body for permission to do the proposed work.
4☐ Ensure that you and the person you're surrogating for maintain your focus and stay present.

Now you can use the pendulum with another person to do anything that you would do for yourself. The pendulum's responses will be the unconscious communications of the other person.

If you suspect that your child has a sensitivity to dairy products, for example, use the pendulum to find out (see the example that follows).

Example:

1☐ You do the pre-tests and corrections on yourself.
2☐ You do the pre-tests on six-year-old Alice, asking her to hold the switching points with her free hand while you hold her other hand with one hand and the pendulum with your other. You instruct Alice to make any necessary corrections.
3☐ While holding Alice's hand you say: *Do I have permission to be a surrogate for Alice?* [The answer is YES.] You hold Alice's hand throughout the procedure.
4☐ You ask: *Do I have permission to find out about Alice's food sensitivities?* [The answer is YES.]
5☐ With the pendulum swinging on the YES/POSITIVE axis, you ask Alice to pick up a glass of milk with her free hand.
6☐ The pendulum immediately changes its swing to the NO/POSITIVE axis.

7□ You ask Alice to put down the drink. Deliberately, you set the pendulum swinging on the YES/POSITIVE axis again. You ask Alice to imagine drinking the milk. The pendulum swings to the NO/STRESSED axis. This is confirmation of Alice's sensitivity to milk.

8□ You go through the same procedure with cheese. Alice again proves sensitive.

9□ You repeat the process with goat's milk, and do not find any sensitivity to goat's milk.

10□ You repeat the process with goat's cheese – which also proves to be okay.

11□ You say: Would it be useful to establish maximum consumption of goat's milk per day? The answer is YES.

12□ Using the methods of calculation with the pendulum from exercises 2.1 and 2.2 you establish that Alice should consume no more than one small glassful of goat's milk per day. Cow's milk and cheese is to be avoided.

Surrogate testing is a wonderful way to help others. It saves time teaching someone how to use the pendulum, and allows you to work with young children and people who, for any reason, are unable to communicate verbally. As a surrogate, you can do everything with another person that you can do on yourself.

However, don't use the pendulum to determine facts – such as which child is bullying your child at school. The pendulum is a fantastic tool for therapy; it's an unreliable tool for judicial enquiry. That way, you'll keep faith with it and achieve amazing results.

Surrogate work can also be done effectively with animals, I am told.

The next chapter begins with a recap of the pre-tests.

4
Essential Tools
for Self-kinesiology

The procedures in chapter 2 are essential to ensure that the pendulum delivers accurate information. It's imperative to make a habit of using these checks. If you don't, you simply won't know whether your results are accurate.

Here is a summary of the pre-checks. These are also available as an appendix. Note that, if you prefer, you can do all the pre-checks using the IC (indicator change) mode in place of the standard +/– mode. The only thing that matters is that you're clear about what you're doing.

Exercise 4.1: Pre-checks

1☐ Start with the pendulum swinging on your YES axis. Zip up the central meridian. If the pendulum swings to NO, make the correction. Zip down the central meridian. If the swing does not change to NO make the correction. Correction: flush by zipping up and down the meridian or use the harmonizing posture.

2☐ Check for switching.
(i) Hold the K27s (the points just beneath the clavicle on either side of the sternum) with a neutral touch. If there is a swing to NO, make the correction. To correct: place a hand over the navel and massage the K27s.
(ii) Hold the ends of the central and governing meridians (just below your bottom lip; under nose) with a neutral touch. If there is a swing to NO, make the correction. To correct: hand over navel and massage just below your bottom lip and under nose.

(iii) Hold the end of the coccyx. If there is a swing to NO, make the correction. To correct: hand over navel and massage tip of coccyx.

3☐ Check for hydration. Say: Water. If there is a swing to NO, drink a glass of water and recheck.

4☐ Check for balanced ionization. Hold one nostril closed with a neutral touch and breathe in and out through the open nostril. Repeat, swapping nostrils. If there is a change to NO, correct by breathing in through one nostril and out the other; do the same with other nostril. Repeat until the check is clear.

5☐ Check for hyperstress. Use IC mode (through intention) and hold your palm upwards. Say: *My body is receptive and amenable to change.* If you don't get an indicator change, place a hand over your forehead very gently and hold until you get an indicator change. Repeat the test.

Troubleshooting

At any time during the pendulum session, if you are getting confused, contradictory or inexplicable results, take the following steps:

1☐ Recheck the central meridian. Stressful issues can cause over-energy in the central meridian, leading to utterly meaningless results.

2☐ Make sure you're clear in your own mind what you want.

3☐ Check that you have permission to do this work. This is particularly important when dealing with areas that your unconscious may not be happy about you looking in to. If your unconscious doesn't give you permission, it won't give you meaningful answers. So leave it alone. Find out what you can do. By doing what your unconscious does permit it is highly likely that eventually you will have permission to address what you're not yet ready for.

4☐ If you think you're getting the answers that you want rather than the truth, apply the pendulum mode.

Having already performed the pre-checks, you are now assured of reliable results and can begin to explore. If you previously dowsed or used a pendulum, you will find – providing you follow the guidelines – that your results are now more reliable and accurate.

Kinesiology corrections

In the pages and chapters that follow you will learn many kinesiology techniques, called *corrections*, which help to overcome stress and bring balance and health. Performing them is beneficial in itself. They will be the beginning of your repertoire of techniques, or corrections, which you will be able to apply to any goal or issue as part of what is called a balance – a term used in kinesiology to refer to a therapeutic session.[1]

It's important that you perform the corrections as you go along, so that your body learns and understands them. Your body will then have a clear idea which corrections will be most beneficial when working with any particular issue.

In this chapter and the next you will be introduced to 11 fundamental kinesiology methods and corrections. Each method or correction and corresponding test (where applicable) is numbered (# 1, # 2, and so on), so that you can readily find them in the text. At the end of chapter 5, the conclusion of part I, is a table of the methods and corrections so far encountered.

Not all the numbered corrections in this book are from kinesiology. There are other effective techniques and methods, from Neuro-linguistic Programming (NLP) and Emotional Freedom Techniques (EFT),[2] for example, to help you to resolve your issues. You'll find an index of all the methods and corrections in the appendices.

The corrections can be applied to any issue. Even corrections which do not appear to have any direct connection with a problem often provide a key to its resolution. So don't omit or dismiss any correction with the thought that it won't be helpful, because it's likely that it will be helpful – if not with the current issue, then with another.

---

1   The idea is that the body's energies are being balanced, as under-energies and over-energies are corrected, thereby restoring the body to health.

2   EFT does derive from kinesiology, but most EFT practitioners are not kinesiologists, and most kinesiologists do not use EFT.

Auditory perception

The first correction (# 1) improves hearing and listening and is often very helpful for people who turn their head frequently in their work. It can also benefit people with dyslexia. Indeed, it can help anybody, including children, to comprehend what they hear more easily.

The correction also helps to facilitate comfort and ease of movement, particularly in turning the head in response to sound, but in fact in relation to any range of motion of the body. If your body is stiff, or certain movements are inhibited, this correction may help.

1 TEST
Auditory perception

1☐　Make sure your body is in a good posture. Start with the pendulum swinging on your YES axis.

2☐　Turn your head to the left. Note the pendulum swing. Turn your head back to the centre.

3☐　Turn your head to the left again, a little further. Note pendulum swing for each turn of head.

4☐　Turn your head to the right. Then back to the centre.

5☐　Turn your head further to the right.

6☐　Now look straight ahead.

If there is a change to NO/STRESSED in any of the above positions, make the correction. Like most kinesiology corrections, the result feels great too! It does no harm to do the correction – and this applies to virtually any kinesiology correction – even if your body hasn't indicated that it is required.

1 CORRECTION
Auditory perception

1☐　Turn your head to the position where you registered a change of pendulum swing, maintaining good posture.

2☐　With your head in that position, reach the opposite arm over your head to your ear. For example, if your head is turned to the left, stretch your right arm over your head to your left ear (it's also okay to use your left hand).

3☐ Unfurl the outer edge of your ear, all the way round, from the top of the ear to the ear lobe. You'll be tugging and massaging the ear outwards, pulling away from the centre of the ear and back towards the head (figure 4.1).

4☐ Repeat (1) to (3) with the head in all the positions that registered a signal change.

5☐ If you have a signal change when looking straight ahead, either (1) simply unfurl both ears; or (2) ask the pendulum (using YES–NO director): *Should I unfurl the right ear?* And: *Should I unfurl the left ear?*

6☐ Recheck the original positions, which should now test clear (i.e. no change of swing should register when the head is turned in these directions).

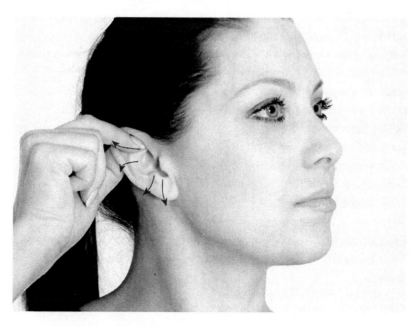

Figure 4.1 Auditory perception correction

Visual perception

The next correction is for visual perception. You will look in all directions, including into the distance and behind you, and note if there is a problem with any view.

Tip:

Move your arm into a position where you can see the swinging pendulum. For example, if you're looking upwards, lift the arm holding the pendulum high up, so you can see the pendulum in your peripheral vision.

2 TEST
Visual perception

1□   With the pendulum swinging on the YES axis, look straight upwards (keeping the head reasonably still). Keep your eyes in this direction and note if there is a signal change.
2□   Now do the same with all the following eye positions, noting all eye positions which produce a change.
3□   Look upwards to the right.
4□   Look upwards to the left.
5□   Look sideways to the right.
6□   Look sideways to the left.
7□   Look straight downwards.
8□   Look down to the right.
9□   Look down to the left.
10□   Now look straight ahead into the distance.
11□   Look straight ahead close up (no more than a foot or two away).
12□   Look in a mirror (but in the distance, not at yourself – which is another story!)

If there is a signal change in any eye position, go to the correction. There is a choice of three corrections to make. One or other or all three corrections are likely to help. The eyes are associated with the kidney meridian in traditional Chinese medicine, and the first correction involves massaging the ends of the kidney meridian. The second correction involves massaging reflex points associated with the kidney meridian. The third correction involves stimulating the points on the head associated with the visual centres of the brain.

The technique given in the correction below invites you to touch the correction point to see whether the correction will help. If touching the point produces an indicator change, that correction is beneficial.

2 CORRECTION
Visual perception

1□   Holding the pendulum where you can see it out of the corner of your eye, look in the direction that caused the change of swing. (As before, you'll probably get a signal change.)

2□   Keep looking in that direction as you (neutral) touch your K27s (see figure 4.2, page 70). Note whether you get a signal change while touching these points.

3□   Looking in the problem direction, firmly touch (with two fingers) one of the two occipital eye points on the back of the head. You will find them on the flat section of the bone just above the ridge at the bottom of the skull above the neck a couple of inches or so from the midline (see figure 4.2). Note whether you get a signal change while touching this point.

4□   Still looking in the problem direction, firmly touch (with two fingers) the anterior deltoid muscle on the upper arm at the front of the shoulder (see figure 4.2). Note whether you get a signal change while touching this point.

5□   A signal change for any of the above means that the problem will respond to the implied correction. Now you know which correction(s) will resolve the problem, here's what you do:
(i) Firmly massage the pair of points that produced a signal change, while looking in the direction that produced the signal change (see figure 4.2). If more than one set of points led to a signal change, massage each pair of points in turn while looking in the same direction.
(ii) Circle the eyes as smoothly as possible, clockwise and anti-clockwise, while massaging the correction points. Again, if more than one correction point indicated, do a clockwise and anticlockwise circle with your eyes while massaging each of the points in turn. You can do this all quickly.

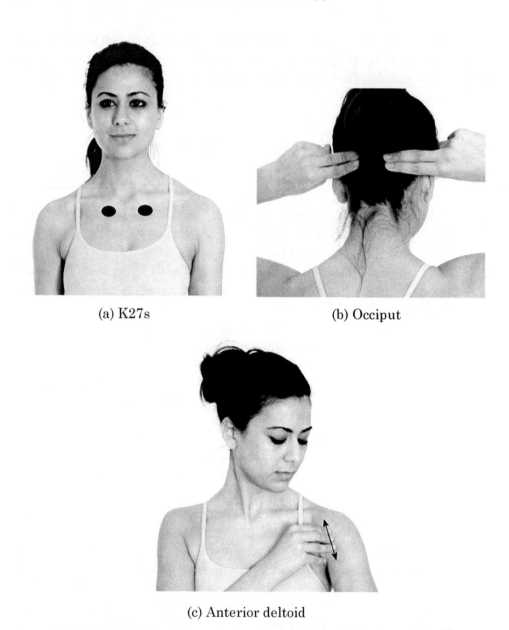

(a) K27s   (b) Occiput

(c) Anterior deltoid

First, massage the correction points while looking in the direction that produced the signal change.

Second, massage the correction points while rotating the eyes (that is, keep your head still and look round in a big circle).

Figure 4.2 Eye correction points

(iii) Recheck that the eye position is clear (i.e. no signal change while looking in that direction).

(iv) Repeat steps (i) to (iii) for each of the eye positions that caused a signal change

Finding the priority

It can be very useful to find the priority when presented with a choice. In the visual perception test above, for example, you may have had more than one eye position indicating a correction, or more than one correction indicating as helpful. The concept of priority can identify the priority issue and the priority correction.

You can find the priority in either of two ways: (1) verbal questioning; or (2) a finger mode.

(1) Verbal questioning

To consider the visual perception correction above, look at the following examples. You would use IC mode.

Example A:

If there were several eye directions that caused a signal change, you can find which eye direction is the priority. You would ask (for example): *Is looking up to the right the priority? Is looking sideways to the left the priority?*

Example B:

Up-right eye position requires a correction. While looking up-right, the points on the occiput and on the shoulder were both indicated as beneficial correction points.

To find the priority correction, ask: *Are the occipital points the priority?* If you get a YES, do them first. If not, ask: *Are the shoulder points the priority?* If so, do them first.

After doing the correction you can look in the direction that caused the signal change and, if there is no change, you know that correction was enough. If you still get a signal change, perform the other correction.

It is more elegant and economical to find the priority since very often correcting the priority makes the other corrections more effective or even unnecessary.

When you want to work with a number of different issues, it can be very helpful to find the priority. Resolving the priority issue first can make it easier to resolve the other issues. Indeed, sometimes your body requires you to address a particular issue before you can resolve others. To find the priority issue, just ask: *Is this the priority issue?* If you get a no for each on the list that you are presenting, check if there's something more important that you need to do first.

It's important to respect the judgement of your body. Sometimes you may decide to do something contrary to what the pendulum tells you. You're going to eat that chocolate or make that commitment or do that business deal even when your body tells you not to. That's fine. That's your (conscious) choice. Just don't fool yourself or try to make the pendulum give you the answer you want. Remember, if your body appears to be giving you contradictory or non-sensical responses, do the pre-checks again. Check the central meridian and check for switching. Check also for hyperstress. Make sure you have permission to do what you're attempting. It's not always granted.

A§ **(2) Finger mode**

Instead of asking for the priority verbally you can use the priority finger mode. To hold this mode, put the tip of your middle finger to the inside crease of the joint in the middle of your thumb (figure 4.3). If you get an indicator change, you have found the priority. The example below shows how it works.

Example:

Your body has indicated two corrections for an eye position, occiput and K27s. Both corrections would be helpful. You want to find out which is priority using the finger mode.

1   Look in the problem direction. The pendulum will give you a signal change.

2   Keep looking in the same direction and touch either one of the eye points on the occiput firmly with two fingers. The pendulum gives a signal change (indicating this is a helpful correction).

3   Still looking in the same direction and touching the eye points on the occiput, put on the priority mode. True, this is a bit tricky while holding the points, but you can do it (you will need to touch the points on the occiput with the ring finger and little finger). There is no signal change. That means this correction is not the priority correction.

4   Still looking in the same direction, touch the K27s firmly. The pendulum gives a signal change (indicating this is a helpful correction).

5   Still looking in the same direction and touching the K27s, put on the priority mode. Again, this is tricky but possible! Now you get a signal change. This means that this correction is indeed the priority correction.

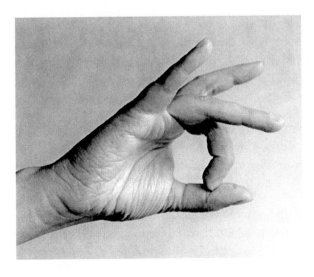

Figure 4.3 The priority finger mode

6   You make the correction and recheck the eye direction. There's no signal change. This means that you don't need to do the occiput correction.

7   If there is a signal change, check which of the remaining corrections is now the priority.

I recommend you practise using the priority mode until it becomes familiar to you. The principle is simple. If you put on the priority mode and get an indicator change, this is the priority.   A§

A§ **The more modes**

Sometimes after doing the corrections, when the original problem is rechecked, there is still a signal change. This means you have helped, but there is more to do. So the question is, does the body want (1) more of the same; or (2) something different? A finger mode can be used to determine this. (Equally, you can just ask; you don't need to use the finger mode. Simply say: *Does my body want more of the same? Does my body want more of something different?* Finger modes simply provide a convenient alternative.)

To find out if your body wants more (i.e. further corrections relating to the issue you're working on), the forefinger and middle finger are placed at the side of the top joint of the thumb (see figure 4.4). If the pendulum registers a signal change, the body is asking for more of something.

To find out if your body wants more of the same correction you were doing, just take the middle finger away, leaving the forefinger there. An indicator change with your forefinger on the side of the thumb means more of the same.

To find out if your body wants more, but of a different correction, replace the middle finger to the position it was in and remove the forefinger. An indicator change with your middle finger on the side of the thumb at the edge of the thumbnail means your body wants more, but of a different correction.

If the eye position still produces a signal change when rechecked, it means that the issue hasn't yet been cleared. Put on the more mode. If you get a signal change, you know the body wants more of something. See if it wants more of the same by using the more of the same mode (forefinger on edge of thumbnail). If that produces a signal change, repeat what you were doing. If it doesn't produce a signal change, try the more of something different mode (middle finger on edge of thumbnail).

As yet, of course, you don't know anything different to do – but you understand the principle. Generally, your body will try to make a successful correction using the information you know, so it's unlikely at this stage that your body will be asking for more of something different. But if you've come back to this after having read and practised other sections of the book, your body may be asking for something else which you now know how to do. If that's the case, ask your body if it wants any of the corrections you've subsequently learned (such as tracing the lemniscate, described later in this chapter).   A§

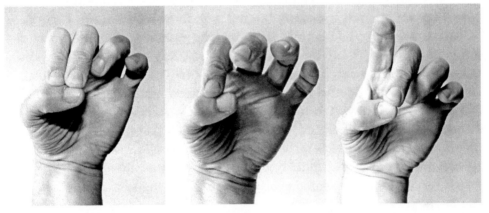

(a) More of something   (b) More of the same   (c) More of something else

Figure 4.4 The more modes

Cross-crawl

This exercise (figure 4.5) helps to integrate and coordinate the left and right brain hemispheres. The left hemisphere of the brain controls the right-hand side of the body and vice-versa. Problems of brain integration can lead to dyslexia, fatigue and lack of coordination.

Sometimes, under stress, a person can flip into one hemisphere or the other and become over-analytical and nit-picky (left-brain dominance) or very emotional, tearful or overwhelmed (right-brain dominance).

The exercise works by encouraging the left and right hemispheres to work together to coordinate movement. By deliberately moving an opposite arm and leg together and by crossing the midline of the body, you are activating both hemispheres of the brain and encouraging them to coordinate their operations. This stimulates the neural pathways of the corpus callosum, the thick bundle of nerve fibres which conducts information between the left and right hemispheres of the brain.

Walking and running are natural cross-crawl activities which many of us do not engage in as often as we should! Walking while carrying an item such as a case, with a rucksack slung over one shoulder, or pushing a pram (as, at time of writing, I have spent much time doing) inhibits the swing of the arms and interferes with the cross-crawl function.

The cross-crawl exercise is simply a matter of walking – or marching – on the spot, very deliberately swinging the left arm forward when the right knee is raised, and very deliberately swinging the right arm forward when the left knee is raised. It can be helpful if the arm that swings forward crosses the midline of the body. In other words, for example, when the right knee is raised the left arm should swing not only forward but over to the right side of the body. The forward-swinging arm can either swing high into the air, or swing gently over the midline for the hand to touch the opposite raised thigh. (See figure 4.6 for additional variations of the cross-crawl.) This exercise should not be performed quickly but, rather, consciously and deliberately. It can also be done in a seated position – raise the thighs and make sure the shoulders are swinging.

The more difficult this exercise is, the more you need to do it!

Before learning to walk, babies usually learn to crawl, involving the co-ordination of left and right sides of the body. Children who don't properly master this important stage can develop dyslexic difficulties later. For anyone with dyslexia, cross-crawl can be particularly beneficial when practised regularly (along with the corrections for switching – especially massaging the K27s). But everyone can benefit from cross-crawl activity. (Figure 4.5 also shows homolateral movement, which is discussed below.)

If you ever get inappropriately tired from walking even just a few steps, or from climbing a few stairs, it may be that brain integration is impaired and your body is working according to a homolateral pattern. The cross-crawl is also very useful if you have been reading or studying for a while and your concentration is flagging or you are tired.

The brain integration test (# 3) checks if your brain is functioning homo-laterally – which would reveal that your left and right brain hemispheres are not presently coordinated. This is remedied, at least temporarily, by cross-crawl. (Later, when working with issues, you may find that the cross-crawl will help address a specific issue or incident.) If all is well, when you look at X there will be no signal change. (A signal change suggests a problem.) However, if all is well, you normally would expect a signal change when look-ing at | |. (No signal change may suggest a problem.

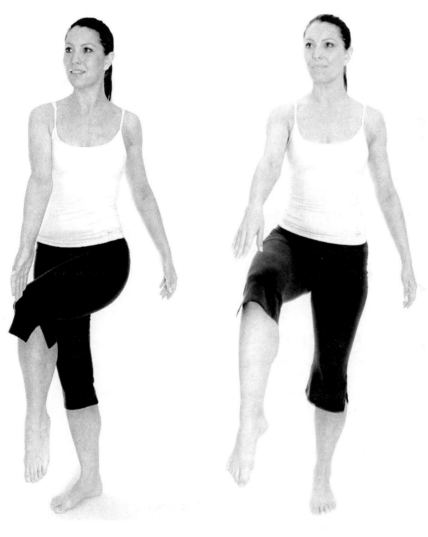

(a) Cross-crawl   (b) Homolateral movement

Figure 4.5 Cross-crawl & homolateral movement

3 TEST
Brain integration (cross-crawl)

1□   Draw a large X on a sheet of paper. On another sheet draw two vertical parallel lines | |.

2□   After doing the pre-tests, put the sheet of paper with the large X roughly at eye-level and take a look at it. (Make sure you're not straining your eyes in any way.) Note whether you get an indicator change.

3□   Put the sheet containing the vertical parallel lines comfortably at eye-level and take a look at it. Note whether you get an indicator change.

4□   If you get an indicator change when looking at X, go to the correction. (If looking at X produces an indicator change you will probably – but not necessarily – have had no indicator change when looking at | |.)

Even if you don't need to do the cross-crawl right now, it might be helpful to spend thirty seconds practising it for future reference. If you need the cross-crawl correction, it may well be that a homolateral action – where the arm and leg on the same side of the body move together – feels easier or more natural (the | | would have produced no signal change). For this reason, the brain integration correction starts with homolateral movement. Changing from homolateral to cross-lateral (cross-crawl) movement and vice-versa helps the brain to be versatile and able to switch from left-brain or right-brain activity to the other hemisphere and to use both hemispheres simultaneously.

3 CORRECTION
Brain integration (cross-crawl)

1□   Begin by marching on the spot using a homolateral action. Lift your left arm and left leg (at the knee) together, then lift your right arm and right leg together, and so on – rather like a puppet on strings. Make the actions deliberate and exaggerated. Do this for ten or twenty seconds.

2□   Now change over to a cross-crawl (cross-lateral) movement: lifting an arm and leg from either side of the body together and allowing the arms to cross over the midline. You can either touch the left thigh with the right hand and the right thigh with the left hand; or you can swing the arm across the body up into the air. This movement should be controlled and deliberate. It is important that the shoulder itself swings (which it will do naturally if the whole arm is swinging – it's no good simply bending the elbow). Maintain this for at least thirty seconds; longer if required.

3□   Repeat (1) and (2) at least once more. Be sure to end with the cross-lateral action.

4□   Repeat the brain integration test above. There should now be no signal change when looking at the X.[3] If there is still a signal change, repeat the brain integration correction and finally repeat the brain integration test.

5□   Ask your body if it is useful to repeat this exercise regularly. If so, find out how often, when and for how long (see the tip on page 81 below).

For most people the natural action is cross-lateral, but tiredness, dehydration or other factors affect brain integration causing homolateral functioning. For a minority of people homolateral movement seems more natural. This is generally a disadvantage (since most activities require both brain hemispheres to work together) and is worth the effort to correct regularly.

If homolateral movement is more natural you may even find any activity involving the integration of both sides of the body tiring and stressful. Walking forward may weaken such people and produces a stressed response; walking backwards often produces an unstressed response.

There are additions to and variations of the correction which may be helpful. The additions involve use of the eyes during cross-crawl (# 4); the variations are of the cross-crawl action itself (figure 4.6).

---

3   There is some controversy in kinesiology circles as to whether or not we should respond adversely to homolateral activity and the two parallel lines. Some people may do work (or sport such as cycling or fencing) where they operate homolaterally. It may not be helpful to them to respond adversely to the parallel lines test or homolateral marching. (However, Gordon Stokes and Daniel Whiteside, in Three in One kinesiology Concepts materials, state that if the indicator muscle remains locked when testing both parallel lines and the crossed lines, this reveals a personality that needs to be in control and always be right. If your testing gives an unstressed response for both, you might want to consider whether this is true for you, and what you want to do about it.)

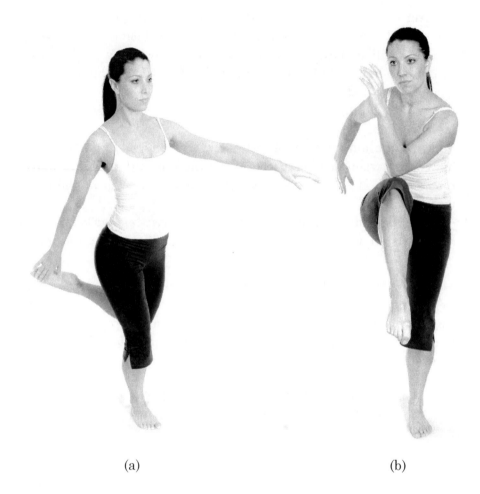

(a) (b)

Figure 4.6 Cross-crawl variations

Notes:

In (a) the hand touches the opposite heel of the lifted foot behind the person while the other arm swings up or across the body.

In (b) the torso twists and the elbow touches the opposite raised knee; the arm and shoulder then swing back and, as the arm swings back, the elbow is brought up to shoulder height but the forearm drops down and back. This movement is believed to benefit the heart.[4]

4 In kinesiology the muscle associated with this movement, subscapularis, relates to heart meridian.

4 CORRECTION
Brain integration (cross-crawl) with eye movements

There are three variations of this correction:

1☐ Perform the cross-crawl while looking at the X that you marked on a sheet of paper.
2☐ Perform cross-crawl while moving the eyes to follow the path of a lemniscate (the infinity symbol, see the next section).
3☐ Perform cross-crawl while deliberately moving your eyes in all different directions.

If cross-crawl with eye movements comes up as a correction, ask the pendulum if it would be most useful (1) to look at X; (2) to follow the path of a lemniscate with your eyes; or (3) to look in different directions randomly while doing the cross-crawl.

Tip:

With any correction, you can find out whether it would be useful to repeat it. Using indicator change mode, ask your body:

1☐ *Would it be useful to perform this correction regularly for a while?* If so: *How often?*
At least once a day/ twice a day/ etc.
At least every other day/ every three days/ etc.

2☐ *Does it matter what time I perform the correction?* If so: *When?*
   (i) *According to* clock *time* (a specific time of day)? If so, find out at what time(s). Or:
   (ii) *According to* event *time* (a time related to a specific activity, such as after eating, after exercise, getting home from work)? If so, find out which activity.

3☐ *For how long do I need to perform the correction?*
For at least one week/ two weeks/ three weeks (and so on)?

Remember to ask these questions again at the end of this period. You may no longer need to perform the correction at all; or the frequency may change.

Tracing the lemniscate or 'lazy eights'

The lemniscate is the infinity symbol, or the figure eight lazily reclining. Like most of the other corrections in this section, tracing the lemniscate is often used in educational contexts to enhance learning and help overcome dyslexic tendencies by encouraging the integration of both cerebral hemispheres.

There are two versions of tracing the lemniscate: the lemniscate for vision and the lemniscate for writing. The procedure for both is similar. There is no specific test to indicate its use but, if reading is tiring, tracing the lemniscate for vision may be very useful; and, if you're having difficulty getting down to writing, then tracing the lemniscate for writing will probably help. Tracing the lemniscate for vision or for writing may also be the body's preferred correction for visual perception (# 2).

Practise each now, and in future simply ask the pendulum if either would be useful.

5 CORRECTION
Tracing the lemniscate for vision

1☐   Extend your right (or dominant) arm out in front of you. In the air, with your forefinger trace the lemniscate, or lazy figure eight, with your fingers, but using large sweeping movements, so that you are moving your whole body as you trace the lemniscates in the air. As you do this, watch your fingers, allowing the head as well as the eyes to move (figure 4.7a).

       Begin by sweeping up-left from the centre; follow the circle down to the left; trace diagonally up and right; follow the circle down to the right; then up diagonally to the left; and so on (figure 4.7a). The lemniscates should always be drawn in this direction because it is the path taken to form individual letters in cursive writing.

       Do a number of these – you can ask the pendulum how many, if you like. Move deliberately, not too fast. Keep breathing comfortably throughout.

2☐   Repeat with your left (or non-dominant) arm.

3☐   Draw lemniscates in the air using both arms, interlocking the fingers but keeping both forefingers straight (figure 4.7b).

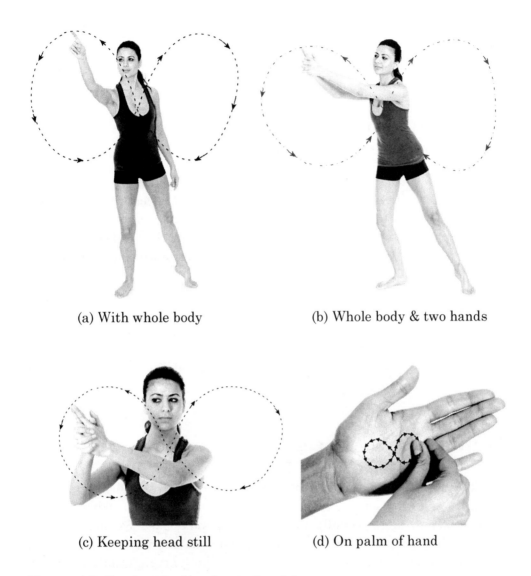

(a) With whole body   (b) Whole body & two hands

(c) Keeping head still   (d) On palm of hand

Figure 4.7 Tracing the lemniscate for vision

4☐ Now interlock the fingers and with both hands trace a smaller lemniscate in the air without involving whole-body movements but keeping the head still and extending the eye muscles. Again, continue the movement a number of times (figure 4.7c).

5☐ With your dominant hand, trace the lemniscate with the thumb, forefinger and middle finger (as if drawing with a pen) in the palm of your non-dominant hand (figure 4.7d). Continue for 20 seconds or so or until smooth.

6☐   Repeat using your non-dominant hand.

6 CORRECTION
Tracing the lemniscate for writing

1☐   On the largest paper you can find (or on a whiteboard or flip chart or similar), draw the lemniscate, filling the whole sheet. Keep your pen or pencil on the paper and continue to draw the lemniscate a number of times – you can ask the pendulum how many times. Make sure your lemniscate always goes (diagonally from the centre) up-and-left and up-and-right.

2☐   Swap hands and repeat.

3☐   Repeat using both hands.

4☐   Now draw a small, individual letter-size lemniscate with one hand and keep drawing it a number of times.

5☐   Draw a small lemniscate with the other hand and keep drawing it a number of times.

Walking freely: the gait reflexes

Walking involves coordination of a number of different muscles to allow the arms and legs to move in the correct time and sequence. When this co-ordination functions optimally, walking is easy and relaxed. But many factors can interfere with physical gait and the symbolic implications of stepping forward. The gait reflexes help to synchronize the synergistic muscles (those that assist the main muscles in walking) and restore coordination, allowing you to tread easily and take the next step – physically and metaphorically.

7 TEST
Gait reflexes

1☐   With the pendulum swinging on one axis, put your hand over the gait reflex points on one foot (figure 4.8) – taking care to retain your balance so you don't accidentally disturb the pendulum's swing.

2⌐ Note whether you get a signal change. A signal change means the correction is required.

3⌐ You can find out which reflex points need massaging by touching firmly with two fingers each correction point (see figure 4.8). A signal change means that point requires attention.

4⌐ Repeat with the other foot.

It doesn't matter whether you want to find out which specific points need massaging or whether you choose to massage them all. The correction (from Touch for Health) is very straightforward.

7 CORRECTION
Gait reflexes

1⌐ Depending on whether you identified specific correction points or not, massage the specific points or all the correction points firmly (they can be very tender).

2⌐ Retest either the specific points (by touching them firmly with two fingers) or putting your hand over all of them. Any signal change indicates that the problem has not yet been completely corrected. If this is the case, try using the more modes (pages 74–5) to identify whether the points need more of the same correction.

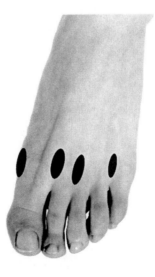

Figure 4.8 Gait correction points

Review

You may have already experienced how working with the exercises in this chapter can make a real difference to how you feel. Ask your pendulum if there are any corrections that would be particularly helpful to repeat right now; or ask the pendulum if there are any it would be helpful to practise again before you continue.

If you are comfortable with the pre-checks and these essential corrections, in the next chapter you can begin to address some of your significant and challenging issues.

5
Relief from Emotional Stress & Distress

Stress is experienced when the demands made of the body are greater than the body's available resources to deal with them comfortably. These demands can be anything and include toxic substances in food, environmental allergies and sensitivities, work pressures, relationship problems, and unresolved traumas from the past. When you experience stress there will be physiological symptoms. The stress will show up as problems in your skin, digestive system, sleep patterns, general health – or any kind of physical disorder.[1] There may also be emotional – often referred to as psychological – symptoms.

A specific form of stress very prevalent in western society is what I call the frustrated fight-or-flight response. In response to perceived danger the body prepares to fight or flee. Blood drains from the thinking centres of the brain as blood is pumped to the major muscles, and cerebrospinal fluid recedes from the frontal lobes to the back of the brain, making rational thought almost impossible. This is helpful if you are confronted by a tiger. If you are in immediate danger it is not helpful to be thinking; urgent action is required – to flee or, if that is not possible, fight. In such circumstances, reconsideration of the meaning and relevance of Hamlet's soliloquy, 'To be or not to be . . .', would be mistimed.

The problem is that the fight-or-flight response is rarely appropriate to the circumstances – it is probably not very often that you are confronted by a tiger or actual physical danger. The 'danger' is more likely to be emotional –

---

1 See chapter 11 for ways of identifying and quantifying these factors in your body.

you are called upon to deliver a public presentation or attend an interview, for example. The most inappropriate action would be to run or fight.

But if you were to fight or flee you wouldn't be in a state of stress; you would be doing what your body is primed for. Stress (that is, frustrated fight-or-flight stress) occurs when the body is on high alert, ready for action, but the conscious mind overrules it and impels it to stay put and be cool. By overruling the body's imperative for action, the fight-or-flight response is frustrated. There is a conflict between the demands of the body, which is prepared for action, and the dictates of the conscious mind, which prohibits action. This is a major stress on the body.

Under these conditions of stress the faculty needed most urgently is not muscle power but the ability to think. But when the body is in the state of frustrated fight or flight, the blood has vacated the thinking areas of the brain, and clear thinking is impossible – the mind has gone blank.

It's not difficult to understand the damaging effects of being in such a state of high alert for any period of time. The digestive organs won't be functioning properly (you don't want to waste energy digesting food if you need to fight or flee – the result is what is often called irritable bowel syndrome, or IBS); the heart and lungs will be working overtime (producing a strain on the heart, inefficient breathing, and a myriad of problems as a consequence); muscles will be tense and flexed (causing discomfort and pain and a physically un-balanced body); and the rational areas of the brain will be sidelined (leaving you unable to think straight).

One way to quickly determine your level of stress is to take a look in the mirror. As you look at your reflection, ensure that your head is upright and your gaze is level: your head should not be tilted up or down. If you see white under one eye, you are suffering from stress. If you see white under both eyes, you are suffering from acute stress. If this is the case with you, take the issue seriously and take action straight away to reduce your stress levels. Why not take a look now?

You can also assess your stress levels using the pendulum. Use the eleven-point scale where zero is completely without stress and ten is the most in-tense level of stress imaginable (see the discussion of subjective units of disturbance below).[2]

---

2   See also # 29 on pages 237–9 to resolve adrenal stress.

There is an effective kinesiology correction which defuses the fight-or-flight response and helps to dispel emotional overwhelm. The correction involves gently holding the two frontal eminences on the forehead – this was the correction for hyperstress (pre-test # 7). These are the two small mounds, prominent more on some people than on others, above the centre of each eyebrow (figure 5.1, page 93). The body knows this correction instinctively. Actors put their hand to their forehead when the character they're playing is under stress. Individuals also do this spontaneously, declaring, *Oh my God!* Parents gently stroke the brows of their children to relax and calm them. I am told that good nurses do this to soothe their patients.

By very gently holding these points you can encourage the blood supply to return to the thinking centres of the brain, quelling the fight-or-flight response and enabling you to think properly again.

Emotional stress release (ESR) to heal past stress

Think of a moderately stressful experience that occurred during the past 24 hours.[3] Choose an experience which, when you think about it, disturbs you in some way and makes you fearful or anxious. The experience may also make you feel (for example) embarrassed, nervous, self-critical or resentful.

Now assess the level of disturbance accompanying the experience. There are three ways you can do this. Try out all three. It might be interesting to compare the numbers you get for each alternative. They may be the same, or it may be that your unconscious body has a different experience to your conscious mind. The first involves your conscious experience; the other two derive directly from your unconscious.

> 1␣ Notice how you feel right now when you think of the experience, and give your feelings a score between zero and ten. (Level ten is the most disturbing you can imagine; zero is no disturbance whatso-

---

3   It might be better not to think of anything too stressful for this exercise if you're still getting used to using the pendulum. If necessary, trace up (there should be no indicator change) and then down (there should be an indicator change) the central meridian to make sure you're getting accurate responses. If the responses are the other way round, do the correction (central meridian flush).

ever.) It's better to get into the experience: be in your own body as you recall the experience (don't watch yourself having the experience or you won't really feel it). This score is referred to as your Subjective Unit of Disturbance (SUD).

2☐ Instead of choosing the number consciously based on how you feel, use your intuition. To do this, simply verbalize the question: *What is the UUD* (unconscious unit of disturbance) *score for this issue?* (Ten is the greatest possible disturbance; zero is neutral.) The answer will usually be the first number that comes into your head (which you will probably hear or see).

3☐ Use the pendulum to find the UUD (exercise 5.1). Don't forget to do your pre-checks if you haven't just done them and to ask permission. Use indicator change mode (IC mode) and YES–NO director (palm mode).

Exercise 5.1: Unconscious Unit of Disturbance (UUD) using a pendulum

1☐   Think of the stressful event and wait until you get a signal change to show that your unconscious has registered it.
2☐   Ask: *What is the UUD level for this event? As much as 1?* (Start at 5 – or any number you like – if you suspect the UUD level to be at least that.)
3☐   If YES, ask: *As much as 2?* And so on.
4☐   Until, for example, you ask, *As much as 6?*, and get no signal change. This would mean your UUD level is not as much as 6, so it is 5.

If there was a difference between the UUD level and your own subjective experience, this may mean that your unconscious body is protecting you from the suffering that your body nevertheless feels. Giving your body a chance to work through the traumas you've experienced, using ESR (and other methods presented in the text) with the pendulum as a guide, will allow you to heal those experiences stored in your body.

Now that you know the level of disturbance, it's time to apply emotional stress release (ESR). It's not usually necessary to test whether ESR would be helpful – unless it is part of a general balance (the term used in kinesiology to refer to a therapeutic session). If you are aware of emotional stress, ESR will almost certainly help.

Tip:

Although I frequently suggest you take a SUD reading, it can also be helpful to take a UUD reading, particularly when you're addressing a past event which doesn't bring up any bad feelings for you on a conscious level.

8 TEST
Emotional stress release (ESR)

1☐ Think about your issue. The pendulum will probably register a signal change to express the stress involved. (If you choose a different issue, take a SUD and maybe a UUD reading.)

2☐ Touch your ESR points. If you get a signal change, do the correction.

8 CORRECTION
Emotional stress release (ESR)

1☐ Very gently touch your 'stress points', the bumps (or frontal eminences) above the eyebrows, with the tips of two fingers of each hand (figure 5.1). The pressure should be just enough to move the skin and no firmer. It is equivalent to the pressure that would be comfortable on your eyelids. If the pressure is too heavy you will be inhibiting rather than promoting the supply of blood to your frontal lobes. You can place your whole hand over your forehead if preferred, or put two fingers and a thumb over the points. The advantage of using the tips of your fingers is that you may be able to feel the pulses (see the tip below).

2☐ While holding the stress points, think about the stressful event.

3☐ Relax, breathe and hold the points for a minute or two, or longer (it can occasionally take as long as 20 minutes to do the job comprehensively), until you feel better, or until the pulses beneath your fingertips synchronize. Stay focused during this time.

4☐ Now recheck the SUD level (or UUD level). It should at least have reduced, and may well be zero.

Tip:

Whenever you are asked to lightly touch points on the head, it will be an advantage if you learn to feel the gentle pulse beneath your fingertips. It may require a bit of practice before you are able to feel the pulses with confidence. It can take several seconds or many minutes for the pulses to be felt at all (if it takes a while you know the correction is particularly beneficial). Ideally, after you are able to feel the pulses, wait until the two pulses synchronize (this can take between 20 seconds and 20 minutes). Once they synchronize, your job is done.

To help feel the pulses, gently tug the skin to one side (or up or down). This aids the process.

But don't worry if you can't feel the pulses yet – with practice you will. A sigh or yawn, or any sensation of energy change, also usually indicates that the job is complete.

ESR to alleviate present stress

The wonderful thing about ESR is that you can apply it to traumatic experiences from the past, stress that you feel in the present, and anxieties you have for the future.

Whenever you feel stressed, simply hold your stress points and breathe. If you can hold these points until you feel the pulses and until they synchronize, you know you have de-stressed your body in relation to this issue.

One useful exercise after a stressful day is to hold your stress points as you review the events of the day backwards, starting from the evening and going through the sequence of the day's events in reverse order. It's great to do this in bed before going to sleep and can help with insomnia.[4]

---

4   Reviewing the day backwards is an idea borrowed from anthroposophy, the philosophy of Rudolph Steiner.

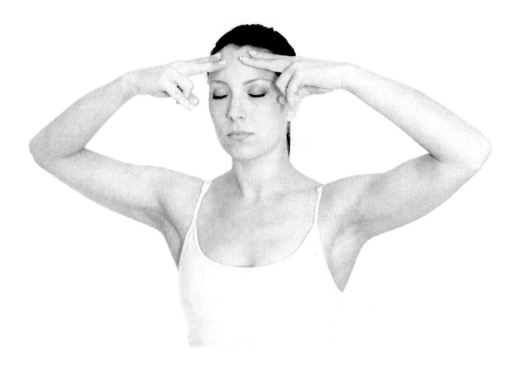

Figure 5.1 Emotional Stress Relief (ESR)

ESR to relieve apprehensions about the future

The procedure here is the same: hold the ESR points while you think about a particular event in the future.

Take a forthcoming event that you feel apprehensive or anxious about. Bring it to mind now. It could be a work event: a presentation; an interview with your line manager; a difficult client; an unpleasant task; reprimanding one of your colleagues or staff. Or it could be something in your personal life: a social event; seeing relatives; meeting someone you're keen on; a confrontation with your children. Take a SUD reading.

Now think through that event as thoroughly as possible while holding your ESR points. (It sometimes helps to be reclining as you do this so your arms don't get too tired and to aid your internal vision.)

Associated and dissociated perspectives

There are two ways that you can think of any event: from an associated and from a dissociated perspective. When you are associated, you are in your body, looking out through your eyes at the imaginary (or remembered) scene. When you are dissociated you are outside of yourself and can see yourself in the picture. It is crucial to think through the anticipated experience from an associated perspective (from inside your body).

It may also be helpful to go through it again dissociated (watching yourself). If you go through a second time dissociated, create a positive picture of how you want to be: watch how confident and at ease you are. Make sure you look exactly as you would like to. When you are happy with what you look like, step into your body again and experience it from the inside. All the time, holding the stress (ESR) points.

When previewing an experience, the more detailed and real that you make your preview, the more benefit you will have when the actual experience arises. You are simply helping your body not to go into fight-or-flight mode during the anticipated event by previewing it in a resourceful state. When the event arrives, your body will recognize it as not being dangerous and you will remain resourceful and able to use your frontal lobes to think and remain in the present.

In the example that follows you are attending an important job interview. You are teaching your body to respond appropriately to the interview, avoiding going into the state of fight or flight. As a result of following the procedure in the exercise, when it's time for the interview, your body knows that there's no threat, and you find that you can continue to think and remain relaxed throughout.

Example:

Imagine you have a job interview next week. You anticipate you'll be nervous the night before, when you're lying in bed ready to go to sleep. Of course, you'll be nervous on waking, and the nerves will stay with you until you leave that interview room.

First, hold your stress points and experience the whole event from the inside, associated. Make sure you fully experience it from the inside. If you begin to see yourself in the picture, step back into your body before continuing. Stay with the feelings that come up, however uncomfortable they are.

You imagine that you're there, lying in bed the night before and eventually fall asleep. You wake up in the morning, have breakfast, and so on. In your imagination you travel to the place where your interview is to be held. You walk in, introduce yourself to the receptionist, sit down, and wait. You listen as your name is called and enter the interview room. You close the door behind you and look at the interview panel. You listen to their questions and you answer with the information you have prepared; and you ask your prepared questions and they answer. You tell them some of your good ideas and they are interested. Finally, you leave the interview room.

You have gone through the entire process from the inside (associated) while holding your stress points. You probably didn't feel confident at all; but that doesn't matter: it was the first time through the experience. It's good to experience the nervousness and acknowledge the range and extent of your feelings. There may also be important things to learn from working through the experience in detail.

Repeat this process a few times, if necessary, until it becomes comfortable and the feelings of fear and stress are completely assuaged.

Now, still holding the ESR points throughout, watch the whole episode from a dissociated perspective. In other words, look at yourself from the outside. But with this crucial difference: watch yourself perform exactly as you would like to perform during the interview: see yourself as happy, enthusiastic, confident, relaxed, and in role. At the end, as you leave the interview, congratulate yourself that it has all gone according to plan.

Repeat this as necessary until you see it all exactly as you would like.

Finally, step inside your body again and experience it from the inside as you behave exactly as you intend. Repeat as necessary.

This is the procedure, while holding your ESR points:

1☐ Experience the event associated, allowing the uncomfortable emotions to be acknowledged.

2☐ Repeat until comfortable.

3☐ Watch yourself from a dissociated perspective, performing exactly as you would like to do.

4☐ Repeat as necessary.

5☐ Step into the picture and, from the inside, experience yourself performing as you would like.

6☐ Repeat as necessary.

You can use the pendulum to check that you have done the job thoroughly. Ask: Are there any parts of the process I need to address more carefully? If YES, find out which parts. Ask: The night before? If NO, ask: On the way to the interview? If NO, ask: When my name is called? And so on, until you get a YES response. (Your intuition might let you know without asking about each section of the process; or you can short-cut the questions by asking, for example: Is it a part before the interview itself? Is it during the interview? And so on.) Then hold your stress points as you focus on the part of the process that indicated. There may have been something you'd forgotten about that your unconscious wants you to be aware of. Then ask if there are any other parts you need to address more carefully. You can also check whether you need to do this process again; if so, how many times and when.

ESR for postural trauma

If trauma to your body occurred when you were in a specific position, it can be very helpful to administer ESR while assuming the posture or body positions of the time the trauma occurred. It is recommended that you have a partner assist you through this process (to hold the ESR points for your while you adopt the required positions).

Example:

Following a car accident in which her car was hit from behind, Angelina still suffers from a neck injury and apprehension when driving – especially when seeing vehicles in the rear-view mirror that are too close to her.

Angelina administers ESR for herself while seated in a similar position to the one she was in when the car was struck. When the pulses synchronize she uses the pendulum to find out if there are other positions which would benefit from ESR.

Angelina found that she needed ESR not only sitting up straight – the position of the initial impact – but also in the positions her body was thrown into during the collision. Angelina's body had first been thrown forward, and then she suffered whiplash when her head was thrown back. She gave herself ESR while adopting each position and checking with the pendulum that she had finished the job.

The SUD value reduced from 8 to 1. Her neck felt considerably better. Although she still felt uncomfortable when vehicles travelled too close behind her, it no longer bothered her in the way that it previously had.

To find out whether ESR would benefit you in relation to a specific event, you can simply ask the pendulum: *Would ESR for postural trauma be helpful?* Then assume the different positions and note whether there is a signal change in each position. If you're unclear what the pendulum is trying to tell you, just ask it straight: *Would ESR in this position help me?*

After doing the ESR, check that the posture is now clear – that is, that the pendulum does not register a signal change. Again, if you're unclear what the pendulum's response means, just ask: *Have I done enough ESR on this posture now?* Or: *Have I eliminated all the stress from this posture?* If you haven't, check the SUD and UUD readings. You might simply need to do ESR for longer (ask the pendulum); or ESR might not be enough in itself. Come back to this experience when you have learned more corrections.

Frontal–occipital (F/O) holding

A variation on ESR holding is to hold the frontal eminences and the occipital lobe at the back of the head at the same time (figure 5.2, page 98).

F/O holding stimulates the visual perception system and enables visual past memory to be accessed and new possibilities to be considered. It also connects the front and back brain, while bringing the body out of the fight/flight response. You are also holding the neuro-vascular reflex points associated with fear (and the kidney meridian).

9 CORRECTION
Frontal–occipital (F/O) holding

1☐   Place one hand very gently over the forehead.
2☐   Place the other on the lower part of the back of the head, over the oc-
      cipital lobe.
3☐   Apply in the same way as ESR.

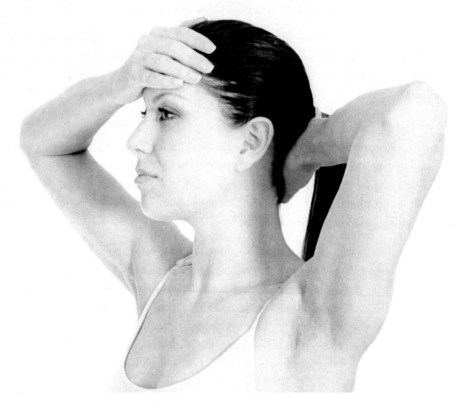

Figure 5.2 Frontal–occipital (F/O) holding

Emotional distress

ESR or frontal–occipital holding will help enable you to eliminate the fight-
or-flight response associated with an incident. Other distressing feelings can
similarly be defused by holding various neuro-vascular points on the head
(figure 5.3).

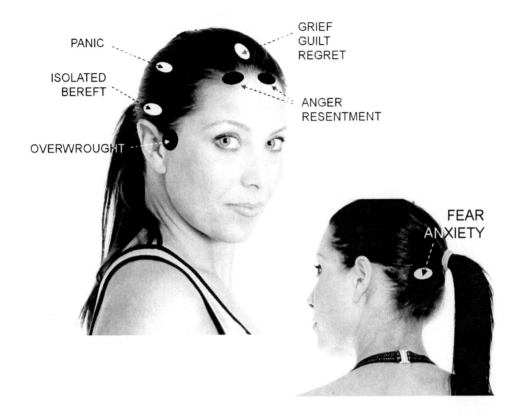

Figure 5.3 Emotional Distress Relief (EDR) neuro-vascular holding points

Note: All points not on the centre-line of the head are paired with a point in the same position on the other side of the head, even if not shown.

10 CORRECTION
Emotional distress release (EDR)

1☐   Do the usual pendulum pre-checks.
2☐   Think of a trauma, or a time that you were criticized, put down, ridiculed or attacked which still distresses you. You will get a signal change from your pendulum as it registers your issue.
3☐   Take a SUD reading.
4☐   Identify the neuro-vascular points and associated emotion. Either:
       (i) Say each stressed emotion from figure 5.3 to yourself (out loud or

silently) and note which emotions give a signal change. Or:
(ii) Touch the points on your head from figure 5.3, and note which one produces a signal change.

5☐   If you get more than one point or pair of points to hold, find out which is the priority. To do this, just ask each, Is this the priority emotion?, or use the priority finger mode (figure 4.3, page 73).

6☐   Connect with the indicated emotion and, with a neutral touch, very gently hold the neuro-vascular points associated with that emotion until the pulses synchronize or until you feel better.

7☐   If there were more than one, check which is the next priority emotion, and hold the points for this. Continue until all the emotions are done.

8☐   Say each stressed emotion (or touch the head points) from figure 5.3 and check they are now all clear (i.e. the pendulum does not respond to any of them).

9☐   Think of the incident or issue you've been working with to check that it is now clear. Re-check the SUD level, which should now have improved. Unless there is more work to be done, there will now probably be no signal change when you think of the incident.

Tips:

• To find out which neuro-vascular points to hold, just touch one of the paired points on either side of the head (there's no need to touch both of the paired points at once).

• For the correction, hold neuro-vascular points very gently – firmly enough to move the skin but with no pressure. The touch should be light enough to be comfortable on your eyelids. Use two fingers for a neutral touch.

• For the paired points (all that aren't on the centre-line of the head), you will need both hands to hold them simultaneously (using two fingers on each point). Feel for the pulses and wait for both to synchronize with each other. If there is only one point to be held (because the point is on the centre-line of the body), still use both hands and hold on either side of the single point with two fingers of each hand, and wait for the pulses beneath both pairs of fingers to synchronize.

Balancing with colour

Colour has a direct effect on the emotions and provides a simple but powerful correction. Each element of the Chinese five-element model (see pages 144 forward) has an associated colour.[5] Looking at one or more of these colours can help to balance the body's energies and heal an emotional issue.

11 CORRECTION
Colour balance

1☐   Think of an emotional issue that you'd like to work with right now.

2☐   Say: *Colour balance*. If this will help, you'll get a signal change.

3☐   Determine whether you need to look at one or more colours at the same time. It's unlikely your body will want to look at more than two at once. Ask: *One colour? Two colours?* And so on.

4☐   Identify the required colours, stating each colour of the five-elements model: *red, yellow, white, blue, green* (a signal change signifies its use-fulness). If none of these colours are indicated (or fewer are indicated than the pendulum suggested you needed in point 3 above), the re-quired colours may not be on the five-element model. Identify them. (*OPTIONAL*: your body may prefer a particular *shade* of that colour. If you have a number of different shades available of the required colour, look at them, and find the one that produces a signal change.)

5☐   Find suitable examples of the colour(s) you need. Make sure the colour(s) are at eye level.

6☐   Apply ESR or F/O holding. Relax and sit comfortably, with full concen-tration, and look at the colour(s), keeping your issue in mind.

7☐   *OPTIONAL*: determine what resolution you would like regarding the issue. Make a statement that describes what you want instead of the issue. Write this down.[6] Say: *Colour balance*. If you get a signal change, the colour balance will help. Proceed from point 3 above, focusing on the resolution statement.

---

5   Table 9.2, page 146. In kinesiology, the water element is associated with *blue*; in traditional Chinese medicine it is more usually associated with *black*.

6   See chapter 12 on how to formulate a goal statement.

		Test	Correction
# 1	Auditory perception	66	66
# 2	Visual perception	68	69
# 3	Brain integration (cross-crawl)	78	78
# 4	Brain integration with eye movements	–	81
# 5	Tracing the lemniscate for vision	–	82
# 6	Tracing the lemniscate for writing	–	84
# 7	Gait reflexes	84	85
# 8	Emotional stress release (ESR)	91	91
# 9	Frontal–occipital holding (F/O)	–	98
# 10	Emotional distress release (EDR)	–	99
# 11	Colour balance	–	101

Table 5.1 Tests and corrections in part I

Self-kinesiology primary balance

Now that your body has experienced many of the fundamentals of kinesiology and knows what happens when these corrections are applied and the benefits they give, you are ready to give yourself a self-kinesiology balance, having available all the corrections encountered so far (exercise 5.2).

Exercise 5.2: Self-kinesiology primary balance

1□   Do the pre-checks.

2□   State your problem or goal. A signal change will register it.

3□   Take a SUD or UUD reading of the problem (either your conscious experience of the problem or an unconscious reading using the pendulum).

4□   Find out which correction is the priority. Using the priority mode, say (or point to) the corrections from table 5.1. If you get a signal change, this correction is the priority.

5□   Once you have done the correction, ask if another correction is required (you can use the more mode), and find the next priority correction. And so on.

6□   When no further corrections are indicated, recheck the SUD or UUD level, which should have significantly improved, and notice how you now feel about your goal or problem.

7□   State the goal or issue again. This time you should no longer get a signal change. If you do, or if you still feel bad about the problem or unconvinced about the goal, you have more work to do on this issue. Come back to it later when you have more tools available.

Part II

CREATING
THE FRAMEWORK

6
The Dawn
of Consciousness

The conscious anomaly

People sometimes express surprise or scepticism about the existence of the unconscious body (otherwise erroneously referred to as 'unconscious mind') – a concept on which kinesiology, NLP, hypnosis and other contemporary therapies depend. But it's not the notion of the unconscious that is surprising; it's the conscious mind that is the anomaly. Think of the animal realm. Apart from human beings, no animal has a conscious mind.[1] But every animal knows exactly how to feed, survive, procreate, and rear its young – and some have highly sophisticated 'cultures'. Animals know what to do because of their unconscious knowledge (not because of conscious thought processes).

Human beings also have unconscious knowledge. We have, in addition, a capacity that distinguishes us from other animals: the conscious mind. It is commonly assumed that it is intelligence that makes human beings exceptional as a species. It is true, our brain capacity is far higher than most other animals. But it is not intelligence that distinguishes us fundamentally from other animals. It is conceivable that an animal of low intelligence could have a conscious mind (though this would be very unfortunate – even if you claim to know a few). It's equally possible for an animal to be highly intelligent but have no conscious mind (some might argue that dolphins are such). What truly distinguishes human beings from animals is a conscious mind, not intelligence. This is the fundamental difference. The greater intelligence

---

1 Even human beings don't start off with a conscious mind, which only develops gradually and is not fully formed until towards the end of adolescence – if it is ever fully formed.

of human beings is only a matter of degree; the conscious mind is a quality of a different order. The conscious mind is the realm of conscious awareness; the arena of thoughts and, to the extent that we are aware of them, perceptions. Animals do not have this conscious awareness.

The question of hegemony

The conscious mind, pretty feeble as its capacities are in comparison with the unconscious body, has however one fundamental advantage: it can routinely override the unconscious in most circumstances. But in matters pertaining to safety and preservation the unconscious body has a much stronger and often overwhelming say. It is fortunate that our preservation is not at the discretion of our conscious mind – or many of us would be unlikely to reach adulthood![2]

In respects other than safety and preservation the conscious mind can easily override the unconscious body; we can go against our nature. This is what willpower means: it is the ability of humans to act contrary to the impulses of our unconscious – our nature. However, the unconscious will attempt to have its opinion felt and we will experience conflict inside ourselves, and slips of the hand or the tongue may occur; or the body may employ other underhand means as it insists on its wishes (the 'Freudian slip').[3] This is the dialectic

---

2   It's because our body responds involuntarily with such vigour to danger that we remain alive. We could easily conclude from this that the unconscious body's first priority is its own preservation. But this isn't necessarily the case. The unconscious is the guardian of our values. There are countless examples of people who have instinctively selflessly risked – and lost – their lives to save the life of another. People also risk their lives for their values. A person's principles (values) can sometimes be more important than his or her own individual life.

3   Freud called this *parapraxis*: slips which reveal unconscious intentions. The unconscious can also take us into madness (which I would see as an enveloping of the conscious mind by the unconscious) as a final resort – which again confirms that it has the final say. (I think this is why Freud preferred the term unconscious to 'subconscious', which implies a hegemony of the conscious mind.) A client once presented to me a very destructive gambling habit and a comparatively defunct conscious mind. The only way his unconscious could prevent him from gambling was to take away his conscious reason. He had tried other measures, but none had worked; so his body was driven to take this extreme measure.

between conscious mind and unconscious body; it is symbolic of the relationship between individual and society. The aim is harmony. When there is harmony there is peace – the achievement of which is one of the greatest aspirations, not only among peoples, but within the individual.

The emergence of the conscious mind

Perhaps at some point in its development the human species had to go against its nature in order to survive. Maybe existence in the forest was threatened and for self-preservation the pre-human species had to come down from the trees and wander on to the savannahs and begin to eat meat. Perhaps this behaviour was entirely at odds with the natural unconscious programme.

In order to go against its own nature – I continue to speculate – the species had to develop another mechanism radically separate from the unconscious programme: one that could react to the exigencies of the moment. The new mechanism would supplement not supplant the old. It would be flexible so that it could change, update and develop – because that's what circumstances dictated. And so the conscious mind evolved, enabling the new individuals to go against their nature and for the first time, as human beings, make deliberate choices. The species of course still needed the unconscious programme to do most of the work. The new faculty would simply allow choice and the ability to supersede the programme.

The birth of the conscious mind is a momentous and defining event: it is the birth of humanity, and therefore of history. Consciousness means self-consciousness, self-awareness, awareness of nakedness. This is the moment of the Fall, of being able to distinguish between good and evil. When human creatures left the forest, they left the Garden of Eden – or they were cast out, fledgling human beings, with new and real consciousness. Not only had human beings self-consciousness (to regard their nakedness) but they had developed the ability to choose.

This is our human destiny, and it is our individual and collective challenge. Choice means freedom and, at the same time, necessarily, responsibility. And responsibility bears the hallmarks of humanity: morality and conscience. An individual's repudiation of responsibility is a repudiation of his or her own humanity.

So the human being stepped out of the Garden of Eden with the newly formed conscious mind and potential for unlimited choice. History begins. And history has primarily been the attempt to justify behaviour – because it must be shown that good was chosen, even when it patently wasn't. Rationality is at the mercy of this drive: to portray the behaviour of one's own tribe as good. However bad the behaviour, one must attempt to persuade others – and oneself – that this behaviour is good, because that is what consciousness demands.

When the pre-human species were simply unconscious, like other dumb animals, they had no choices; they followed their instincts. The ability to choose entirely changes the nature of the beast. Choices have ramifications beyond the individual and what benefits him or her; consciousness of choices entails consciousness of the consequences of choices. Human beings – for that is what the species had become, newly endowed with consciousness – now gained awareness of how their choices benefited others or harmed others. The extent to which an individual's behaviour affects others is the province of morality.

Natural morality[4] concerns the relationship between the individual and others' interests. Others (and their interests) exist in many strata: family, friends, tribe, society, country, continent, world. Conflicts exist within each stratum and between the various strata. Individual morality, which concerns relationships between individuals, is of course very important. The nature and basis of individual morality, I contend, is to make the interests of each individual cohere with the interests of individual others in all strata.

And there is a broader morality too – it is a morality on the social level and defines political parameters. Political morality – the political duty – is to create a world where the interests of any individual are concordant with the interests of all other individuals.[5] This is achieved by fostering institutions

---

4   I am advocating natural morality in contradistinction to religious morality or politically inspired state moralities which maintain absolutes – moral injunctions not based on relationships with other human beings and the consequences of behaviour but on some abstract (and often undisclosed) principle. The purpose of such unnatural 'moralities' is not the benefit of individuals or humankind but the justification of specific behaviour and (probably) the maintenance of control. Natural morality, by contrast, I'm defining as a morality whose principles are based on the consequences of behaviour in relationships with others.

5   This initially involves making the interests of one's own community, region, state, concordant with those of all other communities, regions, states.

and systems which benefit all people. The benefits afforded to any individual through social and political institutions, as far as these institutions affect others, should benefit these others also; at least, these institutions should not be detrimental to others. This should define the political agenda.

Consciousness is an amazing thing in itself. If responsibility is the challenge, there is an upside too. Without consciousness there is no appreciation of the wonders of creation. No beauty. No imagination. No devotion. Consciousness means that human beings are able to construct the terms of their own reality. This is hugely beneficial since it means we can make life better. But it carries responsibility in relation to the lives of others.

The more that human society – that is, its discourses and institutions – evolves, the further human beings are able to stray from their true nature. The demands of the conscious mind easily diverge from the needs of the individual's unconscious body. Society makes demands in contradiction to the demands of the individual's true nature.

The human challenge is to make sense of this contradiction. On an individual level: to live in society while discovering and creating a life according to the individual's true nature. On a social level: to create a society which encourages everyone to be true to their nature.

7
From Feeling to Emotion

The communication of unconscious knowledge

The conscious mind is easily seduced and suborned. Not so the unconscious body. The charming person, the sales patter, flattery can easily deceive the conscious mind. But the unconscious body is alert to everything. The unconscious body knows how to read other people's faces, gestures, smells. It can tell the difference between integrity and superficiality; between real and display; between kindness and deceit.

The unconscious body has had this ability since birth. Since babies are some time from developing a conscious mind, their unconscious responses are unmediated by conscious considerations and the compromises of culture and learned behaviour; their response to other human beings is genuine and immediate.

This is why, contrary to media stories, hypnosis is generally so safe – safer than remaining in conscious control.[1]

Imagine the implications if the conscious mind were able to gain access to unconscious knowledge while awake. This is not only possible, but you already know how to do it: the pendulum provides a way of doing exactly this (but always ask permission).[2]

However, it would be a great advantage to be able to tap into unconscious knowledge without using a pendulum. There is a word for this: *intuition*.

---

1   In hypnosis the unconscious body is foremost and the conscious mind is voluntarily put to the side. The conscious minds of many people can be tricked readily into behaviour that may be detrimental. But the unconscious body – even if it is happy to play along with all sorts of nonsense (as in stage hypnosis) – is far more difficult to fool.

2   Within limits already discussed.

Intuition is about consciously connecting with unconscious knowledge. Being aligned with your unconscious body means behaving in a way that's consonant with unconscious wisdom. This is what is meant by rapport with the unconscious body and is the basis of health and happiness. Your body knows what is good for you and what will make you happy. It wants you to be happy and healthy; it wants to help you to overcome your problems and achieve your goals. All its communications, including uncomfortable feelings, are there to help you and should not be ignored. Your task is to attend to your body's communications with you and trust them.

Of course, your path is not to find out what your body wants in all matters and slavishly follow it. Your challenge is consciously to forge your own path; discover your own adventure; write your own mission. This is your conscious responsibility; but you are entrusted with an unconscious body which will help you to navigate that path.

The unconscious body serves the demands of the conscious mind. It continually gives hints to help in everyday life. Mostly, it operates covertly and with subtlety; this means that the conscious mind is usually able to ignore the directives of the unconscious quite easily. Somatic feelings and their concomitant emotions are the body's primary mode of communication. But much unconscious communication is very discreet: the tiniest inkling that reminds you of something; your eyes looking in an unexpected direction and alighting on an object that reminds you of an activity you need to perform; a tiny thought popping unexpectedly to mind. Mostly people don't give a thought to the source of these subtle communications.

Intense feelings are hard to ignore, but can still be overridden by the conscious will. *The unconscious only intervenes directly under extreme circumstances of emotional and physical threat.*

Trance is the non-conscious state in which the unconscious is in control. Non-hypnotic deep trance states such as shock are the body's way of taking over and protecting an individual from extreme distress. Only if things go very, very wrong do we hear voices or have visions arising from the unconscious. This is not the normal mode of communication of the unconscious![3] For obvious reasons, we need the unconscious to communicate with subtlety.

───────────

3   Indeed, psychosis is hardly a *communication* from unconscious body to conscious mind – it's the unconscious enveloping or subsuming the conscious mind in an act of desperation.

Emotional pain

The conscious mind – the realm of thought – is an autonomous realm. You don't want the unconscious body messing with your head. Fortunately, it usually doesn't. Thoughts are certainly *influenced* by feelings; but conscious control is generally maintained over thoughts. You do not have conscious control over your feelings and associated emotions, but *awareness of your emotions* puts your *behaviour* under conscious control. Where there is a lack of awareness of emotions behaviour tends to be automatic, arising spontaneously from feeling. Unfortunately, this is the rule rather than the exception. The actor of this spontaneous behaviour has no notion that feelings rather than conscious or rational thoughts are their source. Feelings indirectly influence conscious thoughts, since reasons are then provided to explain and justify the unconsciously directed behaviour.

Feelings do not take place in the head and are not inextricably bound up with thinking. Positive thinking, even in the face of adversity, is possible since the conscious mind has its own autonomy and is not at the mercy of somatic feelings; thinking can operate independently of feeling. But this also means that it is possible to ignore, deny and disavow what you feel – which leads to the difficulties.

It is universally acknowledged that physical pain serves an important purpose: that something is wrong and action needs to be taken. Even the painkilling drugs from the pharmacy state on the packet that if the pain persists you should consult your doctor. Without pain you might not bother to take your hand off the stove; you certainly might not be aware the stove is hot. People with leprosy damage themselves by not having such warnings.

Physical pain is the body's red alert (*action must be taken now*); discomfort is amber (*warning*). Whenever the body is in physical discomfort the conscious mind is being alerted to a problem. If something is interfering with the body's ability to heal itself, it is likely that the amber alert will eventually become a red alert unless action is taken.

The mechanism is exactly the same on an emotional level. *Somatic or bodily pain* (since every emotion has a physical corollary) *associated with intense emotional suffering is red alert. Somatic discomfort associated with less intense emotional distress is amber.* The emotional problem will heal by itself, given half a chance. But if this process is impeded, the amber alert is likely eventually to become a red alert.

What are your somatic feelings/emotions telling you? It's actually not that complicated. Empty feelings are saying there is emptiness; lonely feelings are saying there is loneliness; angry feelings that there is anger; and so on. But getting in touch with emotions is something many people have forgotten how to do. How do you get back in touch? It is about *tuning into* the communications your body gives you.

Tuning into the body

The unconscious expresses itself through *somatic feelings*; that is to say, through palpable feelings in the body. This is its general mode of communication: you get feelings in the abdomen and chest (thorax).[4] In English we use the terms *feelings* and *emotions* interchangeably, showing that we (unsurprisingly) unconsciously appreciate their connection. But the two terms are quite distinct in meaning. An *emotion* is an ineffable quality of experience; a *feeling* is its somatic counterpart. All emotions have a concomitant somatic feeling; and all somatic feelings (of this specific type, a sensation in the abdomen and chest) have a concomitant emotion.

First you must develop awareness of these somatic feelings. By *tuning in* to a specific feeling you are able to become aware of the *emotion* that accompanies it. It would be helpful to do this now (exercise 7.1).

Exercise 7.1 Tuning into the somatic feeling

1☐ Think of a situation that makes you feel bad or uncomfortable – perhaps for example when you behaved in a way that you regret.
2☐ Take an initial mental note of the emotion you're aware of.
3☐ Notice where in your body you have the physical feeling. The feeling will be in your abdomen or chest, or perhaps throat. If it's anywhere else it is a *symptom* not a communication. If you have difficulty getting in touch with the physical feeling, relax your muscles and breathe. If you're tense you can't feel. Allow yourself to feel. The feeling might be fairly subtle.

---

4 There may be feelings in other parts of the body too, such as a pain in the back or shoulder – but these are *symptoms* of a problem, not a communication from the unconscious body.

4☐   *Tune in* to the feeling. Notice its quality, size, intensity. Is the feeling a heaviness, a tightness, a pulling, or a churning, for example?[5]

5☐   When you are fully tuned in, become aware of the *emotion* that corresponds with it. (Don't think about it, just tune in. You can't get to it through thinking, only through awareness.)

6☐   Notice that the emotion you are now aware of – which might be difficult to put effectively into words – may be quite different from the emotion that you thought you had before you tuned into it.[6]

If you have any difficulty getting in touch with your feelings, let me reiterate: *you must be relaxed in order to feel.*

Tip:

You need to relax in order to become aware of your somatic feelings. Physical tension prevents you from feeling. To help you to assess the level of tension in your body it is preferable that you stand or lie down. If you are seated it is much more difficult to make this assessment.

If you feel tense, first note the location of tension in your body. Bring awareness and relaxation to these areas. Make sure your abdomen is relaxed and that your abdomen – and not your chest – expands as you inhale. Don't take big breaths, but breathe calmly and easily from low down in your abdomen.

Now it is possible to notice whether you have any somatic feelings in your thorax or abdomen. Tune in. Become aware of the emotion.

Emotions are therefore not the same as *feelings*, although in common parlance the two terms are used interchangeably. Animals have somatic *feel-*

---

5   Resist any temptation to metaphoricize somatic feelings, imbuing them with, for example, a colour or symbolic form. Doing so would be an unhelpful distraction here.

6   Very often the emotion we *think* we have is an extrapolation or deduction from our behaviour or how we think we ought to feel in the circumstances. A person's true emotion only becomes apparent when he tunes into his body. The true emotion may be sadness rather than anger, for example, or fear rather than anxiety.

ings; this is undeniable. But only humans have emotions. To have emotions – the essence of spirituality, the essence of humanity – we need consciousness, a conscious mind. *It is by tuning our conscious awareness in to the somatic feeling that we acknowledge the emotion.* Emotions are not of the conscious mind (they do not equate to thoughts); neither are they of the unconscious body (they do not equate to feelings, or physical body processes). This is why I regard them as *spiritual*; they are the essence of our being because they are unique to *conscious* human beings.[7]

It's now possible to see why some people appear utterly unaware of their emotions. The emotions are clearly deducible by any onlooker because they are exhibited in the person's behaviour; but the person is unaware of them because he or she has not brought *consciousness* (i.e. awareness) to the physical feelings. When people deny the emotions they are so obviously displaying, it may well be that they have no awareness of them.

Denying emotions

Emotions are very often denied, disavowed or renounced. There are plenty of reasons why someone might not want to tune into their feelings and become aware of their emotions. The primary reasons are:

1☐ The demonstration of emotion is a sign of weakness – a crazy but ubiquitous idea, particularly among certain categories of men.

2☐ The expression of emotion, or of specific emotions such as anger or distress, was forbidden or ridiculed as a child. Although the conscious, rational mind may now believe it is acceptable to express

---

7   When René Descartes (*Discourse on Method*, 1637) posed a fundamental distinction between mind and body he made no mention of emotions. Emotions are neither of the mind nor of the body: they are the interface of both. The mind – thinking – for Descartes is the essence of a person. But thought without emotion is like space without stars. Without emotion there is no ethics, no beauty, no love, no freedom, no peace, no happiness. These words relate not to somatic feelings (which we share with animals) but to emotions (which are unique to humans). If Descartes had maintained that emotions are thoughts, this would have been patently false. Emotions presented a double bind for Descartes. He couldn't put them with mind because that would be clearly false (although emotions are often erroneously attributed to mind today); yet he couldn't put them with body because that would separate this vital quality of human beings from what he conceived as the essential self (the mind). So he simply left them out.

emotion, the inhibition is deeply ingrained and the suppression of emotion is habitual.

3☐ There are feelings of guilt or shame about acknowledging certain types of emotion.

4☐ There is a belief that the emotions felt are unjustified and therefore unacceptable. This is probably the most common reason for people to deny their emotions to themselves and others on an everyday basis.

5☐ Some of the feelings stuck in the body are felt as unbearable and better avoided. This is a pattern that may have begun in childhood with dissociation from painful experience. The unbearable feelings are always present in the background, and the sufferer feels there is a constant danger that present emotional upsets will precipitate them. It's considered better to keep the body numb and removed from emotion.

Here is a typical scenario to illustrate the fourth reason, that the feelings are unjustified. You feel hurt and angered by your partner's words or actions but think you *shouldn't* feel this way. Admitting to your feelings would make you feel foolish. Rationally, you believe it's ridiculous to feel so upset (for example) about something so trivial. So you pretend you don't have these feelings. Your partner suspects something is wrong (the unconscious picks up everything) and asks what's up. But you deny there is anything wrong because you disapprove of the feelings and don't want to admit to them. These feelings of upset don't just dissolve into nothing, of course. Indeed, the upset turns into anger towards your partner. But you're hardly aware of these feelings. Later – two minutes later, or next week – you snap at, undermine or attack your partner. Those feelings that you tried to suffocate will find some way to express themselves. Suddenly you and your partner are in a conflict that could have been avoided if only you'd been able to acknowledge your feelings – to yourself, certainly, and preferably also to your partner.

If you protect yourself from emotions for the fifth reason – because the emotions are unbearable – you may well take some form of drugs (legal or illegal, including tobacco and alcohol), or ensure that you keep moving or keep stimulated to help suppress the unbearable feelings. Work on whatever issues your body gives you permission to address. You are very likely to find that, as an adult, acknowledging the feelings that you fear is not nearly as bad as the fear of doing so. This is because, if the experience derives from childhood, *the fear is that of the child.* To the rational mind of an adult the cause of the fear may seem trivial; but to the child it seemed huge. As an adult, you have far more resources to deal with the experience – which is now safely in the past.

Ignoring or suppressing bad feelings is detrimental to health and relationships. If you get into the habit of doing this, emotions become more difficult to recognize or register. The appreciation of pleasant emotions becomes more difficult too, since it is hard to anaesthetize yourself selectively. Though you're trying to ignore them, you still *feel* the bad feelings. They might even be getting worse. You have lost awareness of their *emotional* connection, but the disturbing physical sensation is probably still palpable. You use artificial means (legal or illegal drugs, including cigarettes, alcohol, anti-depressants) to suppress the bad feelings even further. Even good feelings need to be powered by artificial sources (drugs, powerful external stimulation).[8] Eventually, withered inside, life becomes a shadow; the unacknowledged feelings transform into pathology and physical illness.

Men are particularly susceptible to self-induced anaesthesia, since acknowledging certain types of emotional discomfort (such as hurt, pain, embarrassment, self-consciousness, inadequacy, lack of confidence and so on) implies *vulnerability*, while the essence of perceived masculinity is *invulnerability*. Women who occupy positions traditionally assumed by men tend also to be more susceptible to the disavowal of emotions which suggest vulnerability.

Mirrors of experience

The problems founded in childhood tend to play out in later life, demanding resolution. People often think something is wrong with them because they keep making the same mistake. They're right. But, like all problems, by repeating the mistake you have an opportunity to address a problem from your

---

8   Drugs – not least cigarettes and alcohol – are among the easiest and most powerful means of suppressing bad feelings and enhancing good feelings. This is what addiction is all about. But television, music, computer games, avoiding being alone, keeping busy, or eating can also stimulate the senses powerfully enough to mask other feelings that are uncomfortable or painful. Some smokers don't even know what a physical sensation in the chest or abdomen (the somatic communication from the body, as distinct from disease resulting from inhaling the poison) is like. They have suppressed their bodily sensations to such an extent that the only place they can feel is *in the head* – where they're supposed to do their thinking.

past that will change the patterns of your future. Continuing to make the same mistake is a repetition of the same message: you have a specific problem to address.

If you continually choose partners who abuse you, or if you keep encountering bosses at work who manipulate, bully or take advantage of you, there is almost certainly a parallel relationship from the past that is unresolved. By effectively addressing the sources of a problem (which requires more than simply cognitive acknowledgement; specific action is required to *resolve* the past situation),[9] the energy harbouring that problem is released and you can finally steer a different course. Suddenly your next partner treats you with honour and respect. Or suddenly your new boss doesn't try to manipulate you – or your current boss seems miraculously to change.

The principle of projection operates on a social level as well as the personal. For example, white people projected on to brown-skinned people the *discovered darkness in themselves* that they hated and wanted to be rid of: evil, sexuality, primitivity, animality. White Christian morality attempted to exorcise these inherent qualities by projecting them on to black people.

All forms of prejudice are projections of our inner constructions. Imagine how the world could be if we all had the wisdom to know that problems are solved by addressing our own issues and communicating with honesty – as individuals and groups or societies – rather than by attacking other cultures and peoples.

The essence of life

Faced with uncomfortable somatic feelings, and their symptoms and consequences,[10] there are three choices:

1. *Try to ignore the feeling or symptom, hoping it will go away.* The chances are, far from conveniently fading away, it will grow. The fear of travelling on the tube becomes a fear of flying and develops

---

9   Counselling and traditional psychotherapy provide cognitive acknowledgement; but acknowledgement alone is rarely enough to resolve the problem.

10   Symptoms and consequences are what are experienced as the problem, and can include pain in any part of the body; illness; behaviour that is aggressive, suppliant, shy, defensive, apologetic or anything else; addictions and compulsions; fears and phobias; and so on.

into a fear of going over bridges. Or it transforms its nature from a pain in the chest to physical illness, for example.

2☐ *Struggle against the feeling or symptom.* The symptom is designated the enemy. You combat it and strive against it. You harness your resources to quash it. You take drugs, prescribed or proscribed, to neutralize it. But you can never win this fight – even if you remain in the trenches a lifetime. You may even become a martyr to the cause.

3☐ *Acknowledge the feeling or symptom as a friend and ally.* You might as yet have no idea what its purpose is, but you acknowledge that it is serving you in some way and wants the best for you.

The third is the healthy option: the feeling or symptom is there for a good reason.[11] The methods outlined in this book will help you to address the symptom and resolve the cause. (For some problems however you may benefit from the help of a good therapist.)

Without feelings there'd be no action since feelings motivate action. The behaviour of animals and humans is directed by feelings: the behaviour of animals absolutely; the behaviour of humans can be mediated by conscious thought (so that positive feelings direct behaviour). But conscious thoughts and rational arguments are more often used to *justify* actions after the fact than prefigure them.

People who are out of touch with their feelings cannot mediate their behaviour through rational thinking and are governed by their feelings. Such people justify their behaviour with (more or less) rational arguments, and fool themselves into believing that their behaviour has been dictated by their reason – this is particularly (but not exclusively) a male trait and is the basis of nearly all aggressive and destructive behaviour. Although it is widely assumed that behaviour is directed by reason, the contrary is true: behaviour is dictated by feelings and then *justified* by conscious reasoning. *However, if you acknowledge – and thereby take responsibility for – your feelings and concomitant emotions, you are then in a position to control your behaviour.*[12]

Emotions are the essence of life. Without emotions there'd be no concepts of justice, freedom, love, peace, and so on. These concepts would have no meaning

---

11   One of the major presuppositions of NLP (Neuro-linguistic Programming) is that every behaviour, symptom or problem has, or once had, a positive intention.

12   This is discussed in the introduction.

divorced from emotion. We lose sight of the meaning of these words when we lose touch with the emotions that inhabit them. (This is why computers will never be able to *understand*. Understanding – unlike processing information – requires feelings, and feelings require a biological structure.) *Principles and values are given life and meaning through emotion. Divested of emotion, principles and values would shrivel up and lose all meaning.*[13]

Without emotion there is no pain, no heartache, no sorrow. This is true. And without emotion there is no happiness, no joy, no wonder, no beauty, no one-ness. Life is about experiencing the full range of emotions in the present moment. All the emotions are complementary: joy is not possible without sadness; peace is not possible without turmoil; satisfaction is not possible without longing.

Emotions are the essence of humanity and spirituality. They provide direction, purpose, and value. In other words, emotions give life – they are the essence of life.

Uncomfortable emotions are just as valid as the pleasant ones. There are no feelings that are in themselves bad or negative – despite persistent bad press about what are called 'negative' feelings. This attitude helps to create the problem.[14] It is not uncomfortable emotions that require therapeutic intervention but *inappropriate* emotions. Emotions are inappropriate when they have lasted too long or have an intensity disproportionate to what they are responding to.

All experience is emotional. All perceptual, sensory experience has a somatic and emotional component – whether the experience is visual, auditory, kinaesthetic, gustatory or olfactory; and whether the experience is in the present or the recall of memory. Whenever the senses receive information from the outside world, somatic feelings/emotions accompany that information; and when an experience is recalled from memory, there are always feelings associated with it – even if these are subtle. Emotion is an integral part of all experience.[15]

---

13   Beliefs are ideas imbued with feeling; principles and values are particularly important beliefs which are *deeply felt.*

14   The problem is the suppression of emotion.

15   We represent our experience in language. Words only *make sense* (note those terms) because (unconsciously) they evoke past and present sensory experience. This is why words resonate with emotion. Words relate to experience and experience is steeped in emotion.

CENTRAL

Self-respect	*Overwhelm*
Success	*Shyness*
	Shame

GOVERNING

Supported	*Unsupported*
Trust	*Distrust*
Honesty	
Truth	

EARTH

SPLEEN		STOMACH	
Sympathy	*Rejected*	Sympathy	*Disappointment*
Empathy	*Indifference*	Empathy	*Criticism*
Faith in future	*Anxiety for future*	Contentment	*Greed*
Assurance		Harmony	*Disgust*
Confidence		Reliable	*Unreliable*

METAL

LUNG		LARGE INTESTINE	
Cheerful	*Grief*	Self-worth	*Guilt*
Humility	*Depressed*	Letting go	*Grief*
Tolerance	*Haughty/false pride*	Enthusiasm	*Depression*
Modesty	*Intolerance*		

WATER

KIDNEY		BLADDER	
Courage	*Fear/anxiety*	Peace/harmony	*Terror/panic*
Decisive	*Terror*	Patience	*Impatience*
	Careless	Courage	*Fear*
	Reckless	Resoluteness	*Restlessness*

WOOD

LIVER		GALL BLADDER	
Choice	*No choice*	Decisiveness	*Anger*
Love	*Anger*	Love	*Rage/wrath*
Transformation	*Rage/wrath*	Righteousness	*Self-righteousness*
Happiness	*Resentment*	Assertive	*Helpless*

FIRE

HEART		SMALL INTESTINE	
Love	*Hate*	Joy	*Sadness*
Forgiveness	*Anger*	Assimilation	*Overexcited*
Compassion	*Unworthy*	Nourishing	*Discouraged*
Self-worth	*Self-doubt*		
Self-esteem	*Insecure*		
Secure			

CIRCULATION-SEX		TRIPLE WARMER	
Calm	*Hysteria*	Balance	*Despair*
Responsible	*Gloomy*	Elation	*Heaviness*
Relaxation	*Remorse*	Lightness	*Despondent*
Tranquillity	*Jealousy*	Hope	*Hopeless*

Figure 7.1 Five-element emotions

Source: Adapted from Dr Charles Krebs, *A Revolutionary Way of Thinking*, pp. 396–7

Words therefore have a somatic-emotional content since they are evocative of experience and only have meaning in relation to experience. Thought is the realm of the conscious mind and feelings are the realm of the unconscious body. But these two realms are fundamentally interconnected: every thought has some kind of somatic expression. The connection between mind (thought) and body (feelings) is present in every word. This connection is *emotion*.

Involving emotions

Virtually every possible problem or issue – including ones that are apparently completely physical – has an emotional aspect. If we take the emotion into account the work becomes more holistic and the therapy becomes more effective.

Often the emotion will be readily apparent since it is part of the problem. For example, if you were anxious about public speaking, the anxiety is itself the problem. You know already how to tune in to the somatic feelings and acknowledge the emotion (exercise 7.1).

If the emotion is not readily apparent when, for example, addressing physical symptoms during a self-kinesiology session with the therapist within you, identifying the involved emotion helps the kinesiology corrections and other methods to *hold* (that is, to be maintained rather than have only temporary efficacy). Identifying the emotion can also sometimes help to identify the experiences that contributed to the problem and so give you a better understanding of the problem and how to overcome it. Simply identify the involved emotion at the beginning of a therapeutic session to bring it *on line*. Of course, you may travel through a number of significant emotions during the course of a session.

The five-element emotion chart (figure 7.1) will enable you to identify the involved emotion (# 12). Like all the other procedures, this becomes easier and more accurate as your unconscious gets to know the chart better. Take time to look at it so that your unconscious can absorb it. You can identify the involved emotion at the beginning of a self-kinesiology therapy session and at any point during the session when an emotion is required, such as going to an antecedent event in the past. (You will learn the full protocol for a self-kinesiology balance in chapter 13.)

12 CORRECTION
Acknowledging the involved emotion

1☐   Say in turn, or point to, each phase or *element* (fire, earth, metal, water, wood) and central and governing on the five-element emotion chart (figure 7.1, page 124). The one that produces a signal change contains the relevant emotion. (If more than one element is indicated, find the priority.)

2☐   One at a time, say, or point to, each of the meridians of the element. The one that produces a signal change contains the relevant emotion. (Again, if more than one meridian is indicated, find the priority. Have as your intention to find the top priority.)

3☐   Once you have the meridian, go down the list of emotions. The emotion that produces a signal change is the one you are looking for. You can speed up the process by dividing the list into two and saying, *The first half of the list?*, and so on, providing you're clear about exactly what you're referring to.

4☐   Now that you have your priority emotion, repeat the process until you have all the emotions that are relevant (usually one is all that is required).

5☐   State the emotion(s) and let the pendulum acknowledge it by giving a signal change. The emotion is now part of your self-kinesiology balance.

Problems

Past experience governs the response to any new circumstance. The unconscious body evaluates any new circumstance on the basis of past experience (without which the new circumstance would make no sense). When the new circumstance is resonant of past experiences which remain unresolved and cause discomfort, that discomfort is spontaneously re-experienced – although there is usually no conscious cognition of where this discomfort comes from.

These bad old feelings, invoked by new circumstances which are in some way reminiscent of the old unresolved trauma, are what are experienced as problems. These feelings lead you to do things you don't want to do or stop you from doing things you want to do (see the example).

Example:

A new boss reminds you unconsciously of your domineering and aggressive mother. *Towards your boss you behave with passive aggression, having a vague sense of grievance and injustice* – in a very similar way to how you behaved towards your mother as a teenager.

You don't like this behaviour, don't know where it comes from, and have trouble trying to control it. You have no idea you're behaving like an adolescent. Your behaviour doesn't get a good response from your boss, either – which isn't surprising.

The feelings you have when you relate to her are a mixture of anger and fear – which come from an experience at the age of 14 when your mother was furious with you about something that wasn't your fault but you were never given the chance to explain.

People are driven to recreate past scenarios bearing unresolved trauma[16] to give them an opportunity to address and resolve those experiences. By resolving the past trauma the feelings that are at the centre of the problem simply dissolve. Without the interfering feelings you are once again free to behave how you choose.

Bad (i.e. uncomfortable or painful) feelings[17] are an important communication. They are letting you know one (or both) of the following:

---

16   Freud calls this the compulsion to repeat, which he relates to *Thanatos*, the death drive. Transference, the superimposition of a childhood relationship on to the present, is an example of this compulsion to repeat. But the compulsion to repeat is very positive; it has nothing to do with a death drive, in my view. It provides opportunities – as many as required! – to address and resolve the problem, which (until resolved) remains inside the body, draining energy and using up resources.

17   The bad feelings are always there in relation to a problem, but you are not necessarily aware of them. Feelings are dulled when drugs of any kind are taken or if the body is tense. You might be more aware of your behaviour or another symptom of your problem, rather than the feeling. However, your feelings are the key to the problem. This is why it's so important to get in touch with your feelings.

1□ There's something not right in your life at present. For example, you are lonely, overwhelmed, unsatisfied, frustrated, angry.

2□ There's something in your life at present that evokes a past un-resolved trauma. The feelings do not relate properly to the present; they are triggered in the present but derive from a past unresolved trauma.

As regards the first, you don't need self-therapy to feel better. This is not in itself a therapeutic problem. You need (1) to acknowledge the emotion; and (2) to take action to do something about it (such as find a partner; change your job; make new friends; or work less and take more time for yourself). If you have problems making these changes, then you do have a therapeutic problem. Self-therapy may bring temporary alleviation of the bad feelings, but won't provide resolution because resolution requires changing your circumstances.

If your problem relates to the second – a past, unresolved trauma – the action required is to resolve the past trauma, rather than to make changes directly to your life. If you behave badly towards your boss, for example, better to re-solve the problem than try to avoid your boss; or if your problems with your spouse result from issues with your parent, better to resolve that relation-ship in the past than have an affair or terminate the marriage.

8
Past Trauma Resolution

Most therapeutic problems derive from unresolved traumas from the past.[1] This means that something happened in the past that the body wasn't able to process properly, and so the feelings (and emotions) associated with that experience became trapped in the body.[2] These trapped feelings are stirred up whenever something happens in the present that reminds the body of the earlier traumatic experience. The feelings from the source experience, even if they were not consciously acknowledged at the time, are brought into play again.

The key to resolving such problems is therefore to identify and resolve the causes or *sources* of the problem – the unresolved trauma from the past. Resolving the past issue is about *processing* the stored emotions.

Learning how to go back in time to resolve the sources of the problem will make your self-kinesiology immensely powerful. Unless you go back to the sources of the problem (the *antecedent events*) you will only be dealing with the *present manifestation* of the problem. If you only resolve the present manifestation the problem may emerge again in the future (perhaps as soon as tomorrow, or even in ten minutes). If you resolve the problem at its source it is gone for good and can't come back again. Identifying the causes is straightforward with the pendulum; and kinesiology provides the tools to resolve them.

---

1   Other problems, resulting from unhelpful beliefs, derive from *parental brainwashing* (where *parental* refers to any primary carer). A few therapeutic problems are a result *only* of confused thinking (most problems involve an element of confused thinking).

2   If the experience and the feelings associated with it had been properly processed, there would be no problem associated with the experience.

Before you go back into the past, you ask permission. If you are not granted permission there is likely to be corrections you need to perform in the present. Frontal–occipital (F/O) holding while focusing on the present manifestation, or on the antecedent events if you are aware of them, will be very helpful.

The body will not take you anywhere you are not yet ready to go and so, in a problem with a number of antecedents, the pendulum may initially take you to secondary experiences which need to be tackled before you are ready to tackle the primary experiences. It is important to trust your unconscious body and to do what the pendulum suggests. As noted earlier, the body will not be cajoled into doing what it's not prepared to do. The entire point of self-therapy – of any therapy – is to work *with* your body.

The times in the past that you will visit are the times you are ready to visit, and you will visit the antecedent events in the optimum order for your specific issue. This means the pendulum won't necessarily rush you to the primary underlying cause of an issue first. Indeed, there might be quite a bit of work to do before you're ready to address the primary event (if there is such). Patience is essential, and trust that your body knows what's best for you.

Method # 13 is a protocol for identifying and resolving past traumas. The pendulum will direct you to the past issues relating to the problem. Potentially, the most difficult part of this exercise is ascertaining the relevant information at the antecedent age and relating it to your issue (# 13, point 9). Sometimes it is easy to do both; sometimes it's difficult to do either.

To help you to find out what's going on, use your intuition (i.e. the promptings of your unconscious) to come up with ideas, and test them with the pendulum. Keep asking whether you need any more information. If you have trouble remembering anything relevant, ask your body if it is necessary to recall the event. If it is, narrow down the possibilities and make guesses, rejecting or ratifying them with the pendulum. Keep going until the pendulum confirms that you have all the requisite information. Bear in mind that this may not be the only relevant antecedent experience and may not be the most significant. It will however be the most appropriate one to visit at this time.

If nothing comes up at all, check the central meridian. If you really can't come up with anything, ask your body if you can proceed without conscious recollection. When you have all the information you need, ask if you are ready to make the correction. Then find out what correction(s) are required. You will be administering the corrections to your younger self.

The connection between your issue and the antecedent event will very often – but not always – be clear. If you can, make the connection. If you can't, you will still be able to resolve the issue.

By healing your younger self, you are resolving the problem at source. Of course you are not changing the actual events, but it's not the actual events that are significant right now: it's the unprocessed trauma trapped in your body that's creating the problem. This method is so powerful because healing the past trauma ensures that there will be no manifestations of the problem in the present or in the future. This isn't sticky plaster, remedial therapy; this is complete healing.

13 CORRECTION
Identifying the antecedents of an issue

1☐ Think of a problem you'd like to get to the bottom of.
2☐ Do the pre-tests.
3☐ Ask permission to work with this problem.
4☐ Take a SUD reading.
5☐ Determine all the information required about the problem in the present.
6☐ Determine and perform all the corrections required in the present.
7☐ Ask permission to go back in time.
8☐ If permission is granted, go back through the years until you get a signal change. (To do this, see the example that follows.)
9☐ You are now back at a source of the problem. Let your memory and intuition tell you what was going on at this time. If necessary, get help from the pendulum to narrow it down and confirm this is the relevant experience. Determine all the information required about the experience at this time. If you don't make any headway with identifying what was going on, ask if you can make the correction without conscious recall.
10☐ Determine and perform all the corrections required.
11☐ Ask if there are any other past experiences to visit. (You may well have done enough for now.) If there are, find out whether you need to go back further in time or go forward. Then go forward or backwards until you get a signal change. Proceed from point 9 above.
12☐ When there are no more past experiences to visit at this time, ask permission to return to the present.

13☐ Ask your body to return to the present and to give a signal change when you are fully back in the present.

14☐ Take another SUD reading.

15☐ Thank your body for its help.

Example:

To go backward through the years to identify the source of an issue (antecedent event), consider this example of a person who is 35 years old and five months.

A signal change will indicate the involved age. Go back in time in five-year or ten-year segments.

1   *From the present to my 35th birthday.*
2   *34 to 30.*
3   *29 to 20.*
5   *19 to 10.*
6   *Nine to five.* There is a signal change.
7   *Nine.*
8   *Eight.*
9   *Seven.*
10 *Six.* There is a signal change. Six is the relevant age.

Well done. You can now find the sources of any issue. If you wish to, you can take some time now to work on an issue using the protocol above and the corrections you have learned so far.

When you're ready, let's take a look at what energy therapy is about.

9
The Energy of Everything

Qi

The concept of energy, or *qi* (the Chinese term, pronounced *chee*), which underlies kinesiology, is not unique to traditional Chinese medicine. Other non-western traditions have their own conception of energy and their own terms. Even in the West the prevailing science is that energy rather than anything identifiably material is the basis of all things.

The word energy is now permeated with eastern connotations and it's not always clear what is meant by the word. An understanding of the concept of qi is not necessary for these methods to be effective. But perhaps one reason why kinesiology remains relatively little known is that its central concept appears mysterious.

It is true that acupuncture, which is based on the same principles, is very well known; but acupuncture has a long history, while kinesiology is very new. More importantly, acupuncture, like conventional western medicine, is something that is done *to* or *for* (rather than *with*) the patient. The patient of acupuncture doesn't expect to understand its principles any more than the medical patient expects to understand how drugs work.

People who choose kinesiology – and other alternative methods – usually have different expectations: they wish to be *involved* in the treatment. Indeed, kinesiology, interactive in its central principle, *requires* the client's involvement. If the client's attention wanders during muscle testing, the body stops responding (resulting in a *frozen* muscle).[1]

---

1   A frozen muscle is one that remains locked even in response to stimuli which should turn the muscle off.

The problem is that understanding qi is not straightforward. The concept does not derive from western culture, and the medical system to which it refers differs fundamentally from that of western medicine. It is a new concept for most of us. Although there is evidence from different sources for the existence of acupoints,[2] there is no scientific evidence of qi itself. Scientifically, qi remains an inference. Perhaps it is not easy for us to perceive qi because it is integral to the nature of things – in a similar way to how gravity, being integral to our environment, escaped notice for so long before the apple dropped on Newton.

We cannot see qi. However, we can *feel* it. Feeling is not regarded as scientific evidence because it is subjective, and objectivity is the essence of science. However subjectivity, the nature of *experience*, is the essence of human existence.[3]

According to the Chinese tradition we derive qi from: (1) our parents as part of our genetic inheritance; (2) the food we eat; and (3) the air we breathe. The qi from these three sources combine to form the energy that circulates within the body, sustains life and constitutes being. As well as being the vital constituent of life itself, qi facilitates all activity, keeps the body warm, and protects us from disease.

Qi is often thought to be something subtle and insubstantial, and people sometimes ask how something immaterial and invisible can influence the body's physical processes.[4]

But in the Chinese tradition qi is much more than this. Qi is everywhere and in everything. It is not confined to human beings, or even to living organisms; it is integral to *all* things. Qi is the basic constituent of everything. It is not separate from matter; nor is it matter itself. Qi is the quality and character of things; their actuality and their potential. Qi is both state of being

---

2   Acupoints are points on the energy channels of the body responsive to stimulation (using needles or massage, for example).

3   Which is why in so far as psychology is conceived as a science it misses the point: the entirely subjective power of feeling is the force that directs human behaviour.

4   René Descartes grapples with a similar problem after he believes he has succeeded in distinguishing fundamentally between mind and body. How, he asks, can a refined thought actuate the grossest matter?

and process of transformation. Qi is the impulse and life of the universe, connecting everything. Qi is not just the fuel, it is also the engine itself, its motion and power. Energy *constitutes* the body's physical processes; it is not separate from them. *Intervening with the body's energies is an intervention on the physiological, structural and emotional levels, since these are all aspects of energy.*[5]

The energy channels or meridians

Our access to the body's qi (to measure and influence it) is through the energy channels – pathways via which qi is transported throughout the body. The energy channels have three main functions:

1. They are a means of communication within the body – between inner and outer, up and down, back and front – so the body can work as a harmonious whole.
2. They distribute qi to all parts of the body.
3. They regulate and coordinate the functions of the internal organs and glands through the five-element cycles of promotion and control.

There are twelve principal channels, called meridians. Each meridian is actually one segment of a continuous energy pathway that travels around one side of the body, encompassing the front and back of the body, the arms, legs, trunk and head, before looping over to the other side of the body to continue its endless journey (see figure 9.1, pages 136–41).

Each meridian is associated with specific organs or glands in the body and their corresponding functions. The name of the meridian expresses this association. The heart meridian, for example, relates to the heart; the small intestine meridian relates to the small intestine; and so on. The meridians are classified as yin or yang and are associated with a larger unit called an *element,* which informs the characteristics and qualities of the meridian. See the section below entitled 'Five-elements model' (page 144).

---

5   See Ted J. Kaptchuck, *The Web that Has No Weaver* (New York: Congdon & Weed, 1982), for a fuller description of the Chinese conception of qi.

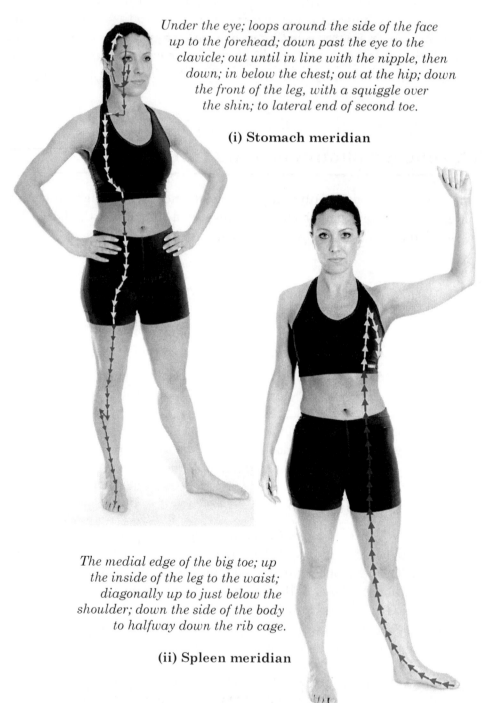

Under the eye; loops around the side of the face up to the forehead; down past the eye to the clavicle; out until in line with the nipple, then down; in below the chest; out at the hip; down the front of the leg, with a squiggle over the shin; to lateral end of second toe.

(i) Stomach meridian

The medial edge of the big toe; up the inside of the leg to the waist; diagonally up to just below the shoulder; down the side of the body to halfway down the rib cage.

(ii) Spleen meridian

Figure 9.1 Meridian paths: (i) & (ii) *(continues)*

Figure 9.1 Meridian paths *(cont'd)*: (iii) & (iv)

Under the armpit; along the underside of the arm and palm to the inside edge of the little fingernail.

(iii) Heart meridian

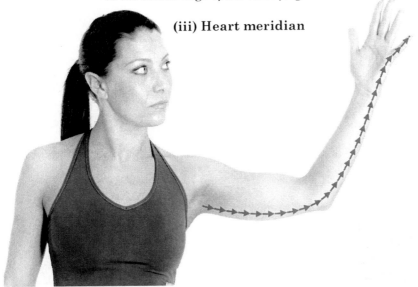

Outside edge of the little fingernail; along the outside of the hand and arm to the back of the shoulder; a few inches down the back; up to the side of the neck; over the cheek to the side of the nose; across the cheek to the ear.

(iv) Small intestine

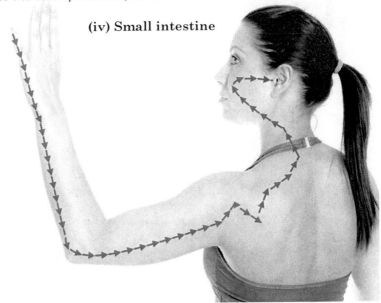

Figure 9.1 Meridian paths *(cont'd)*: (v) & (vi)

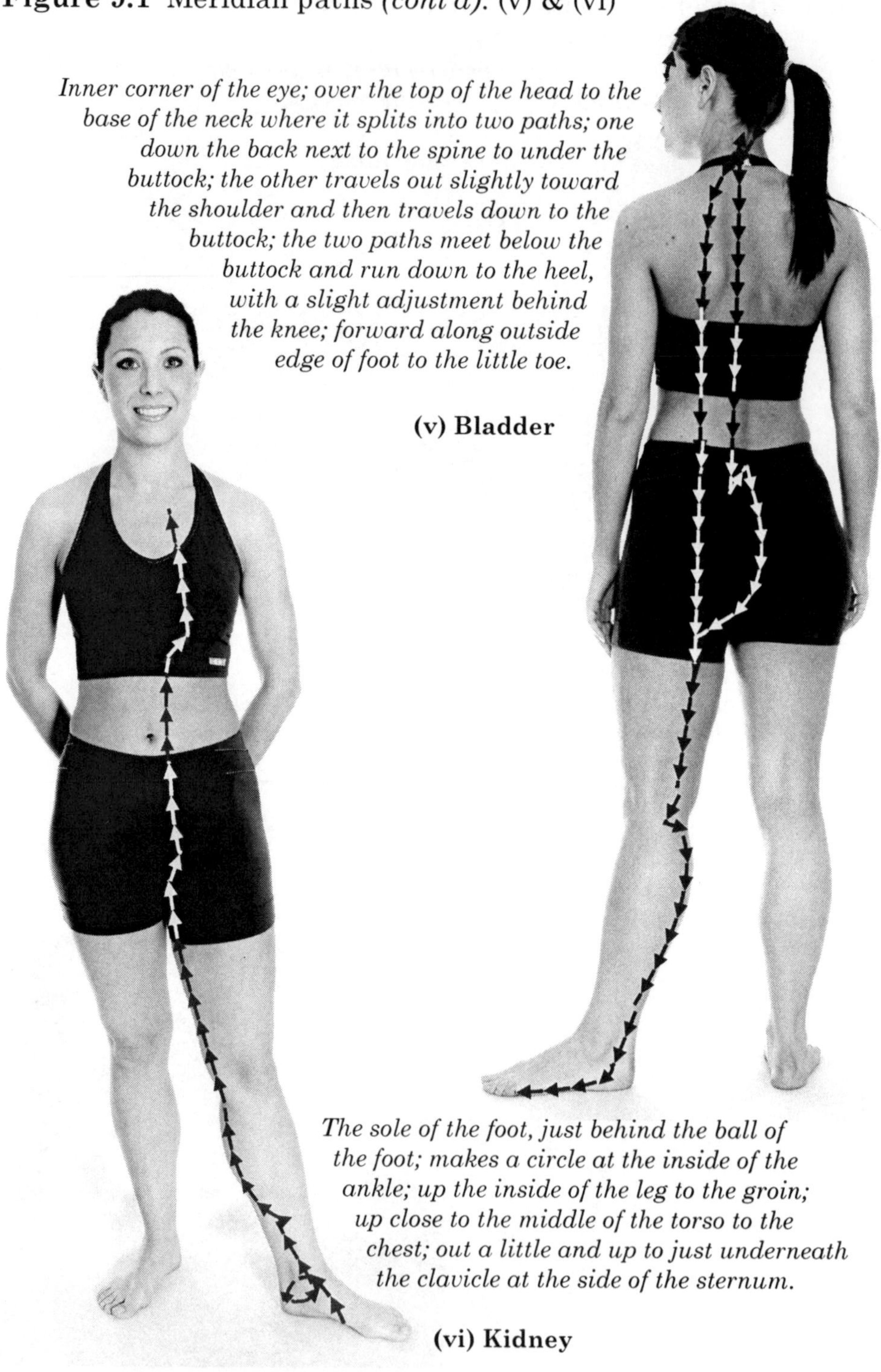

*Inner corner of the eye; over the top of the head to the
base of the neck where it splits into two paths; one
down the back next to the spine to under the
buttock; the other travels out slightly toward
the shoulder and then travels down to the
buttock; the two paths meet below the
buttock and run down to the heel,
with a slight adjustment behind
the knee; forward along outside
edge of foot to the little toe.*

(v) Bladder

*The sole of the foot, just behind the ball of
the foot; makes a circle at the inside of the
ankle; up the inside of the leg to the groin;
up close to the middle of the torso to the
chest; out a little and up to just underneath
the clavicle at the side of the sternum.*

(vi) Kidney

Figure 9.1 Meridian paths *(cont'd)*: (vii) & (viii)

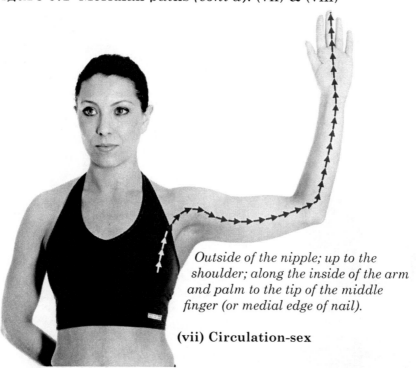

Outside of the nipple; up to the shoulder; along the inside of the arm and palm to the tip of the middle finger (or medial edge of nail).

(vii) Circulation-sex

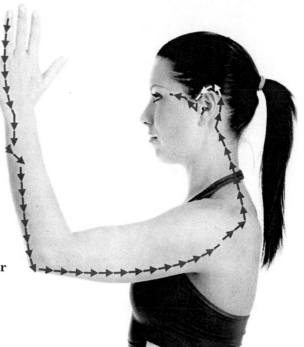

Outside edge of the ring fingernail; up the outside of the arm – with a squiggle just above the wrist – to the shoulder; along to the base of the neck; up and around the ear to the eyebrow.

(viii) Triple Warmer

Figure 9.1 Meridian paths *(cont'd)*: (ix) & (x)

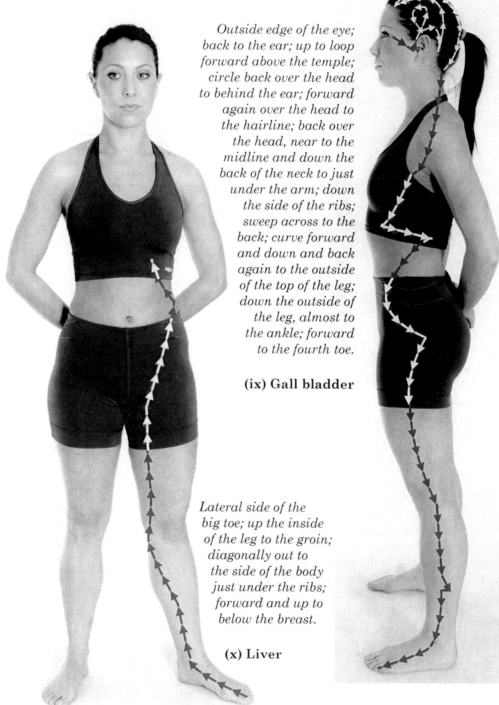

Outside edge of the eye; back to the ear; up to loop forward above the temple; circle back over the head to behind the ear; forward again over the head to the hairline; back over the head, near to the midline and down the back of the neck to just under the arm; down the side of the ribs; sweep across to the back; curve forward and down and back again to the outside of the top of the leg; down the outside of the leg, almost to the ankle; forward to the fourth toe.

(ix) Gall bladder

Lateral side of the big toe; up the inside of the leg to the groin; diagonally out to the side of the body just under the ribs; forward and up to below the breast.

(x) Liver

Figure 9.1 Meridian paths *(cont'd)*: (xi) & (xii)

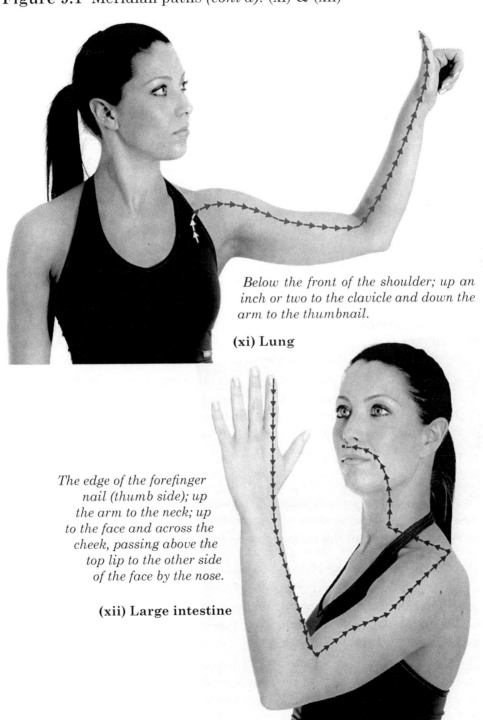

Below the front of the shoulder; up an inch or two to the clavicle and down the arm to the thumbnail.

(xi) Lung

The edge of the forefinger nail (thumb side); up the arm to the neck; up to the face and across the cheek, passing above the top lip to the other side of the face by the nose.

(xii) Large intestine

	Yin	Yang
Fire	Heart	Circulation-sex (pericardium)
	Small intestine	Triple warmer
Earth	Spleen	Stomach
Metal	Lung	Large intestine
Water	Kidney	Bladder
Wood	Liver	Gall bladder

Table 9.1 The five elements and their meridians

What we normally refer to as the meridian is only one segment of the energy channel associated with its particular organ. This is the segment which travels close to the surface of the skin and is accessible to needling or palpating, for example. There are other branches of the meridian that reach deep into the body and connect with the organ associated with the meridian and to the organ of the other meridian of the same element. For example, the lung meridian (the yin meridian of the metal element) runs from just below the shoulder to the thumbnail; this is the part we have access to and refer to as the lung meridian. However, another branch of the channel descends into the large intestine (the yang meridian of the metal element) and comes up again, through the diaphragm, and connects to the lungs.

In addition to the twelve meridians there are many other energy channels. These have functions which include providing reservoirs for surplus qi; supplementing and enhancing communication between the twelve meridians; and carrying qi to parts of the body not served by the twelve meridians.

Apart from two of these channels, most kinesiology systems take little or no notice of the additional channels. These two channels, the central and governing meridians, are ones you have previously encountered. They serve as reservoirs of energy for the other meridians, providing extra qi when required and taking up the surplus qi from the twelve principal channels. The central meridian is associated with the brain; the governing meridian is associated with the central nervous system and the spine. Together, these two channels, though connected to the twelve meridians, form an independent and separate circuit.

The expression of health

Qi travels continually in one direction through the channels. The flow of qi expresses the health and ill health of the body. Unobstructed, free-flowing energy reflects a healthy body. Problems, ill health and disease are represented by blocked meridians and stagnant energy. Energy blocked in one channel will inhibit the supply of energy further up the flow, causing energy imbalances in the system. If certain meridians are depleted of energy, and this depletion becomes chronic or acute, the related organs and glands become starved of energy and disease may result.

The aim of energy therapy is to promote the unobstructed flow of qi through the meridians, producing balance, which is the expression of good health. To this end, acupuncture uses needles and moxibustion to influence the flow of qi and correct imbalances. Kinesiology has various methods of influencing the flow of qi in the meridians. To facilitate balance, the kinesiologist (like the acupuncturist) stimulates energy flow to meridians where qi is depleted (condition of under-energy) from the meridians where there is too much qi (over-energy). Balancing the meridians in this way improves the health of the body and the functioning of its organs and facilitates healing and optimum performance.[1]

Our energies are said to be balanced when the flow of qi is unimpeded and there are no pronounced over-energies or under-energies in any meridians in the system. Good health equates to a dynamic equilibrium, rather than a completely uniform balance – which would not be possible or desirable since we are living creatures.

With our energy operating within certain parameters – like the low- and high-water mark of the tide – we function optimally. Our energy system is affected every moment by internal and external factors. At different times of the day different meridians become more active (see figure 10.5, the meridian energy wheel). The changing seasons affect the balance of qi. From emotion to emotion the balance changes. Indeed, as we shall soon witness, every emotion that we have changes the energy configurations of our meridians. It is only if this imbalance becomes extreme, or lasts too long, that our health is at risk.

---

1   It is important to be clear that an energy imbalance in a meridian usually does not mean that there is any problem with the associated organ itself.

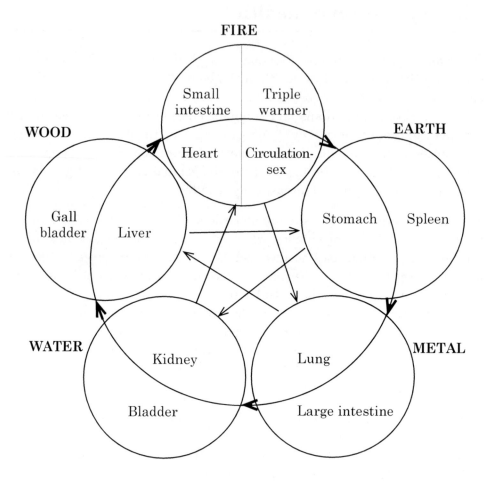

Figure 9.2 The five-elements model

Note: Each element relates to a colour, listed in table 9.2, page 146.

Five-elements model

The five-elements model (figure 9.2) is one of the foundations of traditional Chinese medicine and is fundamental to the conception of energy in kinesiology. The theory symbolically describes the process of change to which *all things* in the universe are subject – including human beings and the meridian system.

Five-element theory not only describes the phases within the body, but the relationship between the body and the environment. The name of the element suggests its characteristics. *Fire* is characterized by heat flaring upward; *earth* by growth and nourishment; *metal* by purification and solidity; *water* by cold and flowing downward; *wood* by germination and spreading out freely.

Each element relates to seasons that have these characteristics: fire is associated with summer; earth to late summer; metal to autumn; water to winter; wood to spring. Each element is also associated with a particular taste, smell, and sense organ. The elements (and their associated meridians) have emotions, sounds and colours connected with them (table 9.2). Individuals are considered to have characteristics associated with one or more elements (my own character relates more to the water element; you might want to consider which element your character relates to).

There are two types of relationship between the elements, creating two cycles: a cycle of promotion and a cycle of control. The cycle of promotion, called *sheng*, is also referred to as the parent–child relationship. According to the five-element model (figure 9.2), this cycle moves in a clockwise direction from element to element: fire promotes earth; earth promotes metal; and so on. Symbolically:

   o   Fire promotes earth by making the land fertile.
   o   Earth promotes metal since metal is formed inside the earth.
   o   Metal promotes water deep in the earth.
   o   Water promotes wood by helping it to grow.
   o   Wood promotes fire as fuel.

The cycle of control, called *ko*, is referred to as the grandparent–child relationship. According to the five-element model each element exercises control over the element two steps ahead. For example, fire controls metal; metal controls wood; and so on. The ko cycle ensures equilibrium and harmony.

   o   Fire controls metal, as fire can melt and mould metal.
   o   Earth controls water, as earth gives water boundaries and keeps it in check.
   o   Metal controls wood, as metal chops and shapes wood.
   o   Water controls fire, as it is able to extinguish fire.
   o   Wood controls earth, as wood grows inside earth.

Through the cycles of promotion and control, which provide checks and balances, the five elements maintain equilibrium. Although, for example, earth controls water, water can indirectly control earth by promoting wood, which can control earth.

And if earth controls water excessively, water is unable to control or constrain fire; fire becomes strong and over-controls metal. Metal cannot therefore constrain wood, so wood increases its control over earth. In this way the whole system maintains a dynamic equilibrium.

	FIRE	EARTH	METAL	WATER	WOOD
EMOTIONS	love joy hate	sympathy empathy	guilt grief regret	fear anxiety	anger resentment
SOUNDS	laughing	singing deep sighing	crying	groaning	shouting
COLOURS	red	yellow	white	blue	green

Table 9.2 Element emotions, colours and sounds

Diagnosing imbalances

The practitioner of traditional Chinese medicine will monitor the radial wrist pulses, look at the hue of the skin, examine the tongue and so on in order to diagnose energy imbalances. Imbalances are then corrected through diet, herbs and, of course, the use of needles to influence the flow of energy in the meridians.

The kinesiologist uses muscle monitoring to determine imbalances, since specific muscles relate to specific meridians. By testing specific muscles, information can be gained about energy imbalances in the meridians. In kinesiology a single indicator muscle can also be used to determine energy imbalances using *alarm points*.

Alarm points

The pendulum, too, can determine imbalances through the *alarm points* (*mu* points).[2] Alarm points are acupoints which provide information about qi imbalances. There is an alarm point for each meridian (figure 9.3, page 148).

Tip:

> Use the pendulum to determine the exact location of the alarm points. You may get a partial signal change (the pendulum swinging at an oblique angle) when you are close to the spot. You will get a full signal change when you touch the exact spot.

By touching a meridian's alarm point we can find out whether the meridian is under-energized or over-energized. If the pendulum registers a change of swing when we touch the alarm point (with medium pressure) we know that there is an imbalance in the meridian. Whether the meridian is over- or under-energy can be determined through the degree of pressure used when touching the alarm point (with two fingers).

- If a *medium-pressure touch* on the alarm point produces a signal change, there is an imbalance in the meridian: it is *either* over-energized *or* under-energized (or possibly both).
- If a very *light touch* on the alarm point produces a signal change, there is *over-energy* in the meridian.
- If a *heavy touch* on the alarm point produces a signal change, there is *under-energy* in the meridian.

Example:

1☐ Touching the lung meridian with a medium pressure produces a signal change. This means that the lung meridian is either over-energized or under-energized.

---

2   *Mu* means to collect. The alarm points are collection points of qi relating to the channel, and indicate deficiency and surplus.

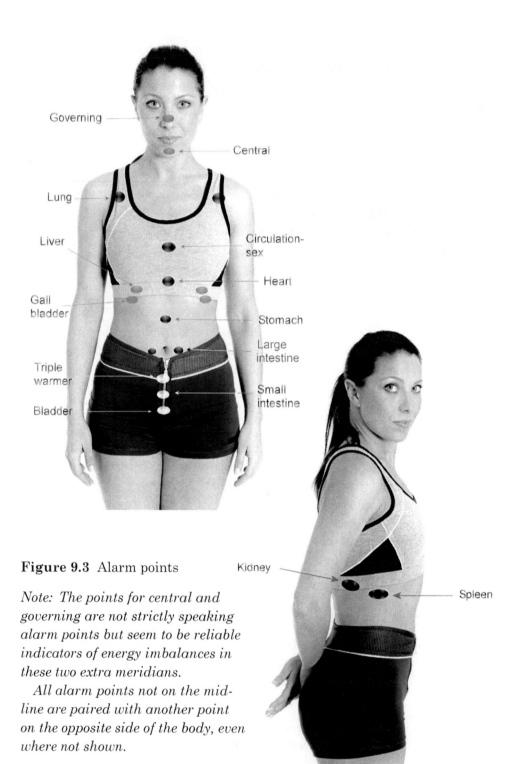

Figure 9.3 Alarm points

Note: The points for central and governing are not strictly speaking alarm points but seem to be reliable indicators of energy imbalances in these two extra meridians.

All alarm points not on the midline are paired with another point on the opposite side of the body, even where not shown.

2☐ Touch with a light pressure produces no signal change.

3☐ Touch with heavy pressure produces a signal change. The lung meridian is therefore under-energized.

It does seem to be possible that, on occasion, a meridian can be at the same time both over-energized and under-energized. So be aware of that possibility. Generally, it is preferable to use a heavy touch, since you will prefer to correct under-energies.

Touching the alarm points with one hand while holding your pendulum with the other can be tricky. Be careful with some of them (notably the alarm point for the kidney meridian) that the movement of your body as you prepare to touch the alarm point does not in itself cause a signal change. If you think that might have happened, simply ask the pendulum to give you another signal change if the meridian is indicated. Do exercise 9.1 to help you to become familiar with the alarm points.

Exercise 9.1 Monitoring the alarm points

1☐ Do the pre-tests.

2☐ Using two fingers, touch each alarm point (on left and right sides of the body) with moderate pressure, noting any signal changes.

3☐ For every alarm point that produced a signal change, test again using a light touch (for over-energy). If there is no signal change, use a heavy touch (for under-energy), which will produce a signal change. Note the results.

Energy configurations

You now have a current reading of your meridians. I'd like you to try something.

Exercise 9.2 Energy configurations

1☐ Choose an emotive word, such as *war, love, sex, politics, God.*

2☐ Say the word and allow the pendulum to give you a signal change to register it.

3☐ Check the alarm points again. Notice that the reading you get may be completely different from your previous one.

How can a word affect the energy system? Words are not just jots of sound or scribble, they are neurologically charged. A word has meaning in relation to all of our experiences connected with that word; it carries with it all the (unconscious and preconscious)[3] memories of its associations. Just saying this word has changed your previous energy configuration.

You might want to do the same thing a second time: check your energy configuration after choosing a different word, or try saying the name of someone who stirs up pleasant or unpleasant emotions in you.

You could choose a less conceptual word, such as coffee, alcohol, cigarettes to test. However, there might be a great difference in your result, depending on whether you are testing the effect of coffee on your system, or your associations of the word. If you just want the associations of the word, say the word *coffee* to yourself and check your alarm points. If you want to find out what coffee does to your energy configuration, have a sip of coffee and then check the alarm points; alternatively, imagine drinking a cup of coffee, and check the alarm points.

After doing this, if you go back again and re-check the first word you chose (in exercise 9.2). You will find that the energy configuration you have now is not the same as it was originally.

The body's energies interrelate with everything that's going on to produce different configurations. This suggests – perhaps unsurprisingly – that all feelings, and the body's energetic expression of them, affect all other related feelings. More reason, if you need it, not to dwell on negative *thoughts*. However, I hardly need to say that it is vitally important to acknowledge your *feelings*.[4]

Renewing the past

Like words, memories and experiences are not static or homogeneous; memories are not fixed in space and time. They don't have to torment you forever.

---

3   Memories that are preconscious are capable of being recollected consciously.

4   It is quite possible (and highly desirable) to acknowledge bad feelings (which are not under conscious control) and remain positive in thinking (which is within conscious control) since, as discussed in chapter 7, thoughts and feelings are separate realms. This is one way that some people who have suffered terribly not only survive but remain healthy and happy.

Problem memories and experiences are emotion-charged interpretations of the past which can be modified in the present – just as the present is modified by the past.

The past, after all, *is only ever a representation in the present*. The past is not real, not any more. Now it's just a figment of your mind and body. You're never actually dealing with the past; *you're only ever working with the present's version – its representation – of the past.*

Armed with the pendulum, you can intervene in the 'past' and transform your experiences and resolve your traumas. That's why it's never too late to have a happy childhood. And that's why, whatever it was that happened, and however awful, you can transform your perception and response to the experience. When it was the present, the past was a reality; it no longer is. You can change it by changing your perception of it or your body's representation of it.

Identifying pronounced imbalances

The alarm points reveal energy configurations in the body which are the expression of immediate concerns. All unresolved issues, including all those not presently in conscious awareness, are expressed in the underlying, essential energy flow. The flow that we read through the alarm points very often do not register the compensations the body makes for longer term imbalances.

This is why it is so important to resolve past traumas. Even when they are not currently troubling you, they are in the background absorbing and depleting your energy. As you know, problems in the present are opportunities to resolve underlying issues from the past. Exercise 9.3 lets you know whether a specific issue results in pronounced energy imbalances.

Exercise 9.3 Pronounced energy imbalances

1☐   Ask the pendulum to register only *pronounced* under- or over-energies. Let it give you a signal change to acknowledge your request.
2☐   Check your energy system *in the clear* (i.e. before introducing any stimulus) by using the alarm points (medium pressure) and the pendulum. You will probably not get any signal changes unless you currently have

       pronounced imbalances. (If you do, don't worry: the corrections in the next chapter should help to rectify them.)

3☐   Take one of the emotive words suggested above, or a different one, and check your alarm points. In all probability, none will produce a signal change – suggesting that the energy fluctuations produced by the stimulus are within an acceptable range (i.e. are not pronounced).

4☐   Think of a significant trauma or issue that you have. Let the pendulum acknowledge it with a signal change.

5☐   Ask: *Do I have permission to use this issue for this exercise?*

6☐   Check for switching (K27s; under nose and just below bottom lip; tip of coccyx); and check the central meridian (zip up and then down). Correct if necessary. (The stress caused by bringing to mind a severe trauma can cause switching and over-energy in the central vessel.)

7☐   Let the pendulum know you only want pronounced imbalances to register; it will acknowledge your request with a signal change.

8☐   Check the alarm points again. This time you may well find one or several meridians with pronounced under- or over-energies.

Of course, the word *pronounced* is completely subjective. If we say that 100 is the optimum energy in a meridian, you can ask the pendulum what deviation it considers unhealthy or pronounced. For me, around 60–65 and below is pronounced under-energy; 128–30 and above is pronounced over-energy. Your scores may be different. Using your score as a reference point can be useful if you want to find out the score value of your over- and under-energized meridians in relation to your own problems and concerns. Doing so would be for interest only. Resolving, rather than measuring, your problems is what's important. However, it is motivating to measure progress made. Measuring the scale of the problem before and after your interventions can be encouraging when the problem hasn't been completely resolved.

Now you know how to get a reading of your meridians. The next thing to learn is how to balance those meridians. In the following chapter you will learn three major energy-balancing techniques: improving lymphatic drainage; stimulating blood flow to specific organs; and tonifying or sedating meridians. By balancing your energies you are balancing your whole system – physiologically, structurally and emotionally – since everything is energy.

10
Lymph, Blood & Energy

When George Goodheart was first developing what was later called Applied Kinesiology, he borrowed and adapted two fundamental pioneering techniques to correct energy imbalances and strengthen muscles. From Frank Chapman, an osteopath, he learned how to improve the functioning of the lymphatic system by massaging what are now known as neuro-lymphatic reflex points; and from Terrence Bennett, a chiropractor, he learned how to encourage blood flow to specific organs by very gently holding neuro-vascular reflex points.

Both of these methods help to balance meridians and are very effective in promoting and maintaining good health and in helping to overcome problems and achieve goals.

Neuro-lymphatic (NL) reflex points

Typically undervalued by western medicine, a properly functioning lymphatic system is crucial to health. There are twice as many lymph vessels and twice as much lymph as blood vessels and blood in the body. Blood supplies the cells with nutrients, and the lymph drains toxins and other waste from the cells and carries them to lymph nodes, where they are digested by lymphocytes (white blood cells). The lymph also transports unused proteins and fats from the tissues for delivery back into the bloodstream. All the lymph is eventually deposited back into the bloodstream near the base of the neck.

Unlike blood, which has its own pump (the heart), the movement of lymph relies on contraction of muscles and fibres stimulated by physical exercise. Oedema (the accumulation of fluid, particularly water, in the tissues) is a result of inadequate lymphatic drainage of the waste products of the cells. This leads to a lowering of resistance to infection and impairs the body's ability to heal.

People with oedema are often chronically dehydrated. The medical practice of prescribing diuretics is counterproductive. The body is trying desperately to dilute the waste products in the excess lymph and there is not enough water in the tissues. If you have oedema, use the pendulum to find out how much pure water you should be drinking, and which neuro-lymphatic points you should be massaging. Bouncing on a trampet or similar as well as general exercise is also very helpful in stimulating lymphatic drainage.

Other symptoms of lymphatic congestion include a string of pearls around the outside of the iris, and swollen neuro-lymphatic reflex points which feel squishy, rubbery, or contain little hard lumps (if the problem is chronic). When the problem is chronic the neuro-lymphatic correction described below may need to be repeated over a considerable time.

You don't have to be ill, of course, to benefit from this correction. Like all kinesiology corrections, it will help to bring your body – and specific energy channels – into balance.

The neuro-lymphatic corrections are often even more effective if muscles are exercised before and after the corrections are applied. It is helpful to test for the correction after doing a particular form of exercise – whether it's walking, gardening, climbing the stairs, cycling, doing sit-ups, lifting an object and so on. Preferably after doing at least a little of a specific physical activity, do the lymphatic reflexes test.

14a TEST
Neuro-lymphatic (NL) reflexes (elements)

1   *Optional:* do a little of a specific physical exercise.
2   Say: *Lymphatic system.*
3   If you get a signal change, you need to find out which neuro-lymphatic reflex points need attention.

4   Say: *Fire; Earth; Metal; Water; Wood; Central, Governing* (see figure
     9.2 on page 144). Pause after each element in readiness for a signal
     change. At least one element will produce a signal change (if more than
     one, find the priority; but if you have in mind that you are looking for
     priority only one should show up). If central or governing produce a
     signal change, go to point 6 below.

5   Name each meridian belonging to that element. The meridian that
     produces a signal change requires the lymphatic correction.

6   You may not need to stimulate all of the lymphatic points related to
     the indicated meridian. Touch the various points. Each one that pro-
     duces a signal change requires the correction.

7   Perform the correction: massage the indicated correction points deeply
     with a neutral touch for between 10 and 30 seconds or until any tender-
     ness has become more comfortable. (See the correction below.)

8   Say the name of the meridian that produced a signal change. If there
     is no signal change, the meridian is now balanced. If you get a signal
     change, there is more work to do on that meridian. Touch the neuro-
     lymphatic points again. Repeat the correction for any that indicated.
     If the meridian still indicates, but no neuro-lymphatic points indicate,
     then another correction is required. Try the other corrections in this
     chapter.

The neuro-lymphatic (NL) correction points are located on the front of the
body, mainly on the chest, abdomen and pubic bone; on the back, mainly
either side of the spine; and on the upper legs (see figure 10.1, page 156).[1]
The points on the back are not easy to touch, and are even more difficult to
massage. If you have a helper, ask him or her to touch, massage and challenge the points for you. If the points are too awkward to reach, make do with
using the ones you can reach.

Like all the other corrections, your body will understand the NL corrections
much better after you have practised them.

At first, your body may not be familiar with the elements. As you work with
them, and with the meridians, your body will become more accustomed to
them and is likely to give you highly accurate readings of the meridians and
elements.

---

1   The NL reflex points shown here are only a portion of the NL reflex points
used in Touch for Health.

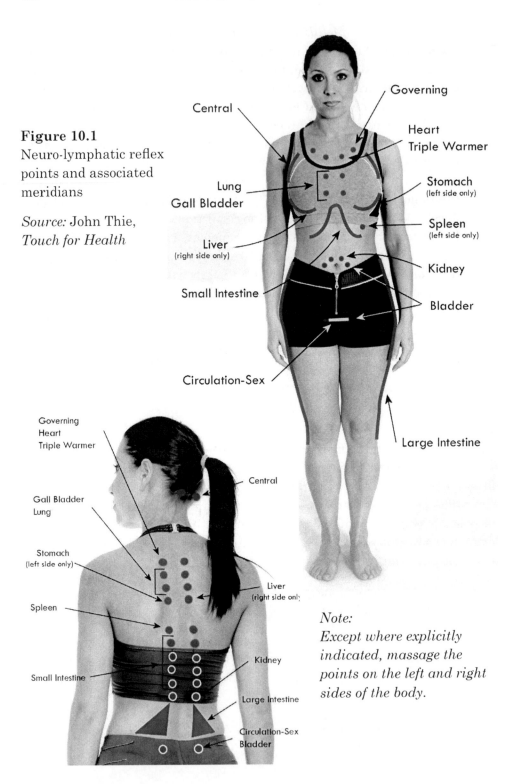

Figure 10.1
Neuro-lymphatic reflex
points and associated
meridians

Source: John Thie,
Touch for Health

Central

Governing

Heart
Triple Warmer

Lung
Gall Bladder

Stomach
(left side only)

Spleen
(left side only)

Liver
(right side only)

Kidney

Small Intestine

Bladder

Circulation-Sex

Large Intestine

Governing
Heart
Triple Warmer

Central

Gall Bladder
Lung

Stomach
(left side only)

Liver
(right side only)

Spleen

Small Intestine

Kidney

Large Intestine

Circulation-Sex
Bladder

Note:
Except where explicitly
indicated, massage the
points on the left and right
sides of the body.

14 CORRECTION
Neuro-lymphatic (NL) reflexes

1   Massage the indicated points deeply for 10 to 30 seconds. If the lymphatic area is greater than a single point, treat it as a series of individual points, massaging one point at a time. If the points are tender, massage more gently for longer. (You can also hold the ESR points – the frontal bone eminences – to alleviate any discomfort; holding the end of the implicated meridian will also help to alleviate discomfort.) The more tender the points are, the more they are likely to benefit from attention.

2   Allow the pendulum to swing on the YES axis in the clear. Using the pendulum, challenge the NL points by touching them firmly while the pendulum is swinging. If there is a signal change, the points need further massage (or another correction – use the more modes in figure 4.4, page 75, to find out); otherwise, your job is done.

3   Optional: repeat the physical exercise and recheck the NL points.

Tip:

To help strengthen your abdominal muscles, after doing sit-ups massage the neuro-lymphatic areas for the small intestine meridian. The front NL points specifically for the abdominal muscles are along the inside of the thigh from the groin area to halfway down the upper leg. There are three vertical bands to massage on the thigh: (1) along the inside of the leg; (2) slightly to the front; and (3) slightly to the back. The NL points to massage on the back are the prominent knobs on the hip bones on either side of the spine.

Sometimes this correction won't 'hold' and, within moments, you're back to square one. To help this correction to hold, it is sometimes useful to take the following steps, which enables cerebrospinal fluid to circulate more easily around the skull, providing energy to the abdominal muscles.

1□   Using all four fingers of each hand and, as firmly as is comfortable, press along either side of the midline of your head and pull apart, as if you are trying to pull apart your skull from the middle. Start at the forehead (just above the eyebrows) and take a controlled breath as you pull both sides of the skull apart.

2☐ Work backward, along the head, in stages. The next position is at the front of the top of the head; then the back of the top of the head; finally, the back of the head. (See figure 10.2.)

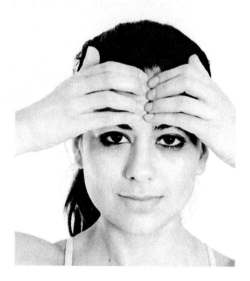

Figure 10.2 Treating the skull for circulation of cerebrospinal fluid

As an alternative to using the elements to find which neuro-lymphatic points need attention, you can use the meridian alarm points (# 14b).

14b TEST
Neuro-lymphatic (NL) reflexes (alarm points)

1　Find the under-energized alarm point (using heavy pressure) (see figure 9.3, page 148). Remember to include central and governing meridians. If there is more than one, find the priority.

2　Firmly touch, in turn, all the NL points associated with that meridian, noting the ones that produce a signal change.

3　Correct by massaging the NL points that were indicated (refer to # 14 correction above).

4   Challenge (by firmly touching one of the reflex points) to make sure it is now clear. If you still get a signal change, massage the points some more, or use the more modes on page 75 (figure 4.4) to find out which alternative corrections the body would now like.

5   Using heavy pressure, touch the indicated alarm point again. This should now be clear (no signal change).

6   If more than one meridian was indicated, find the next priority (if one still indicates) and locate and massage the points associated with that meridian. And so on.

Neuro-vascular (NV) reflex points

The neuro-vascular points, which again have associations with each meridian, are mainly located on the head. Holding them very gently helps to stimulate blood flow to specific parts of the body and benefits the meridian and organ or gland associated with it. You may remember having come upon neuro-vascular reflexes earlier: Emotional Stress Release (ESR) and Emotional Distress Release (EDR) points (chapter 5).

For the correction, the NV points should be held with two fingers very gently – with pressure that would be comfortable on the eyelids. Holding with the tips of two fingers on the point allows you to feel for tiny pulses. Learning to feel the pulses can take a little practice, and sometimes the pulses cannot be felt until the points have been held for a while.

If time permits, hold the points until you feel the pulses under both sets of fingers synchronize. (If you are holding a single, midline point, you can still use two fingers of each hand to hold either side of the point – so you'd have four fingers touching the point – and wait for the pulses to synchronize.) Once the pulses have synchronized, your job is done. This may take between 20 or 30 seconds and several minutes or even longer. It can take as long as half an hour. Even if you don't have time to hold the points until the pulses synchronize, holding them for a shorter time will help. If you can't feel the pulses or are not able to wait until they synchronize, check the pendulum again while touching the same neuro-vascular points to see whether you have done enough. If you have, the pendulum will not register a signal change. (See figure 10.3, page 160.) If there is a change of swing, hold the points for longer (if possible), or see if another correction is indicated.

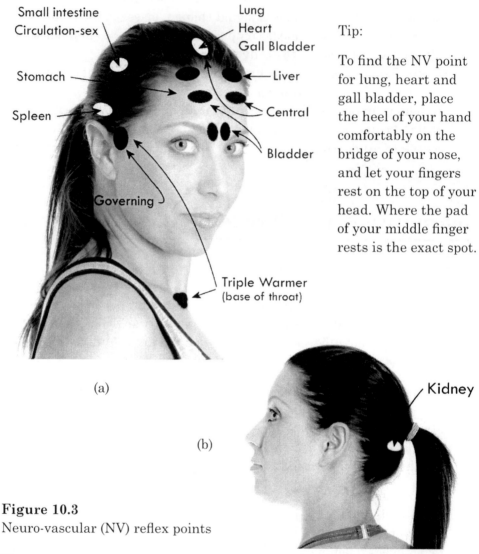

Small intestine
Circulation-sex

Stomach

Spleen

Governing

Lung
Heart
Gall Bladder

Liver

Central

Bladder

Triple Warmer
(base of throat)

Tip:

To find the NV point
for lung, heart and
gall bladder, place
the heel of your hand
comfortably on the
bridge of your nose,
and let your fingers
rest on the top of your
head. Where the pad
of your middle finger
rests is the exact spot.

(a)

(b)

Kidney

Figure 10.3
Neuro-vascular (NV) reflex points

Notes:

All points that are not on the midline are bilateral (that is, they are on both sides of the head), even where only one point is shown, and should be held at the same time. Some meridians involve more than one pair of points.

Balancing the body through stimulating neuro-vascular reflexes is very similar to the procedure for the lymphatic system.

15 TEST
Neuro-vascular (NV) reflexes (elements)

1   Say: *Vascular system*
2   If there is a signal change, find the points which need attention by us-
     ing the elements from figure 9.2 in the previous chapter. State each
     element in turn. The element that produces a signal change requires
     the correction (for example, the Wood element).
3   If more than one element indicates, find the priority.
4   Identify which meridian on that element requires attention by naming
     the meridians associated with the element, noting the one that pro-
     duces a signal change (for example, the liver meridian).
5   Identify the NV points to hold (if more than one set) by touching the
     points on your body (figure 10.3). The ones that produce a signal change
     need attention.

15 CORRECTION
Neuro-vascular (NV) reflexes

1   Hold the NV points very gently, preferably until the pulses synchron-
     ize.
2   Challenge by touching the NV points again. There should be no signal
     change. If there is, hold the points for a little longer (or identify a differ-
     ent correction).
3   Stating the meridian and element again will produce no signal change
     if your work has finished.
4   If more than one element indicated, find the next priority. According
     to the instructions above, identify the meridian that needs attention,
     then the NV points, and do the required correction.
5   Restate: *Vascular system*. There should now be no signal change.

Like the NL points, the NV points can be found through the alarm points.
The principle is exactly the same except that, instead of firmly touching the
NL points you'll be lightly touching the NV points.

Exercise 10.1 shows you how to work with NL and NV points in combination.

Exercise 10.1: NV and NL reflexes

1   Find an under-energized alarm point (using heavy pressure). If there is more than one, find the priority.
2   Firmly touch all the NL points associated with that meridian, noting any that produce a signal change.
3   Lightly touch, in turn, all the NV points associated with that meridian, noting any that produce a signal change.
4   If one or the other (NL *or* NV) has indicated, perform the relevant correction. If both NL and NV have indicated, find the priority and perform the correction. For a NL correction, massage the points; for a NV correction, hold the points gently, preferably until the pulses synchronize.
5   Challenge (by gently touching a reflex point) to make sure it is now clear. If you still get a signal change, check whether the body now requires a NL or NV correction, or use the more modes in figure 4.4 and find the required correction.
6   If a second correction was performed, challenge again, and find another correction if required.
7   Using heavy pressure, touch the indicated alarm point again. This should now be clear (no signal change).
8   If more than one meridian was indicated find the next priority and make the necessary corrections. And so on.

Balancing meridians

The energy system provides a reading of the health of the body; but it is not just a passive *expression* of the health of the body. Interventions can be made directly on the energy system to *influence* the energy system. Creating a more harmonious energetic system, by removing blocks and drawing energy from over-energized channels to those that are depleted, improves overall health.

That is what acupuncture does. According to traditional Chinese medicine ill health is the result of qi blockages and resultant energy imbalances. Needles or moxibustion are used directly to influence energy flow, bringing the body into balance.

You have seen how stimulating lymphatic and vascular reflexes can immediately restore balance to the energy system. Kinesiology also has techniques to intervene directly on the energy system: tracing the path of the meridian (see below); and stimulating acupoints either to tonify or sedate a meridian.

A§ Tracing the meridian energy flow

George Goodheart, the father of kinesiology, discovered that tracing the flow of the meridian with the fingers often strengthened particular muscles. We shall use this technique to encourage energy flow in under-energized meridians. For the meridian paths refer to figure 9.1 (pages 136–41).

16 CORRECTION
Tracing the meridian

1   Do the pre-checks.
2   Check the meridian alarm points using heavy pressure (looking for under-energized meridians).
3   If you get more than one, find the priority meridian (using the priority mode you will get a signal change if it is the priority).
4   Lightly touch the beginning or end of the meridian (neutral touch). If you get a signal change, the correction is indicated.
5   Trace the meridian with a deliberate movement in the direction of the energy flow (using two fingers). It's helpful to make light contact with the body at the beginning and end of the meridian (at least). As you trace the meridian continue to make light contact or keep your fingers within an inch or two of the body. It is not essential to trace the path exactly. Repeat twice more if desired.
6   Touch the beginning or end of the meridian again to challenge. If you still get a signal change, trace the meridian again and challenge again or find another correction.
7   Now recheck the alarm point. It may now be clear (no signal change). If you get a signal change, the meridian needs more attention. Try the lymphatic and/or vascular corrections, as well as the corrections below.   A§

Acupoints to tonify and sedate

These are meridian points which encourage energy flow to a meridian (to tonify) or release energy from a meridian (to sedate). On each meridian there are acupoints which relate to every element. The acupoints to tonify relate to those meridians which feed into the channel; the acupoints to sedate relate to those meridians which the channel itself feeds.

To tonify or sedate a meridian simply hold the two pairs of acupoints sequentially. Holding the first pair encourages more energy into the meridian, if the purpose is to tonify; and encourages energy to flow out of the meridian if the purpose is to sedate (*sheng* cycle). Holding the second pair of acupoints, whether the intention is to tonify or sedate, stabilizes and controls this flow (*ko* cycle).

17 CORRECTION
Acupoints to tonify and sedate

1   Use the alarm points to find *under-energized* meridians (heavy pressure) and find the priority. If either the central or governing meridian is under-energized, use the *central & governing hook up* to correct it (see correction # 18 below).

2   Refer to figure 10.4 for the acupoints to tonify associated with the under-energized meridian. Hold the first pair of acupoints to tonify for 30 seconds or so, or until the pulses under the two pairs of fingers synchronize. You can use the pendulum to check whether you have done enough: either simply ask; or use the more modes (page 75).

3   Hold the second pair for 20 seconds or so to stabilize the flow.

4   Recheck the alarm point by touching with heavy pressure. A signal change means the correction is not enough to balance the meridian. See if other corrections (including neuro-lymphatic and neuro-vascular, outlined above) will help.

5   Find the next priority under-energized meridian and correct in the same way. Repeat until all the alarm points are clear. (Bear in mind that correcting one may automatically have corrected the others.)

6   Now test the alarm points for *over-energy* (light touch). It is most likely that all of these will now be clear. (If so, you've completed this exercise; skip to the end of the exercise.) If there is more than one (which is unlikely), find the priority.

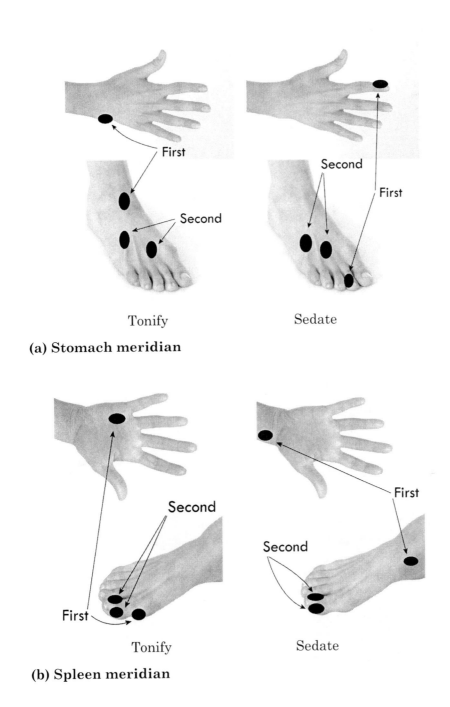

Tonify

Sedate

(a) Stomach meridian

Tonify

Sedate

(b) Spleen meridian

Figure 10.4 Acupoints to tonify and sedate meridians (a) to (b) *(continues)*

Note: Hold both the first points for about 30 seconds; hold both the second points for about 20 seconds.

Figure 10.4 *(cont'd)* (c) to (d)

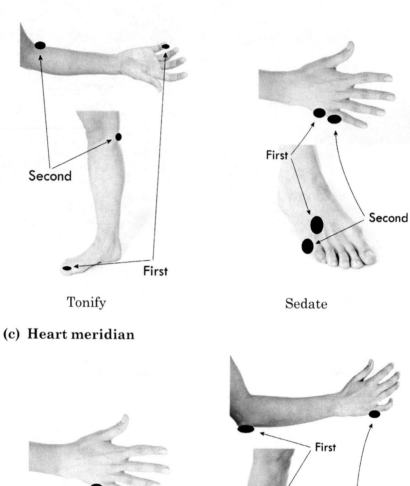

Tonify   Sedate

(c) Heart meridian

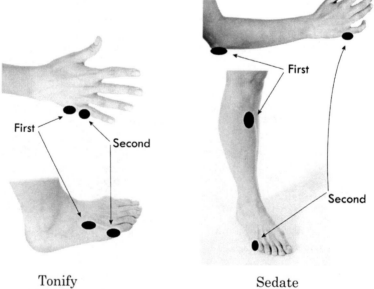

Tonify   Sedate

(d) Small intestine meridian

Figure 10.4 *(cont'd)* (e) to (f)

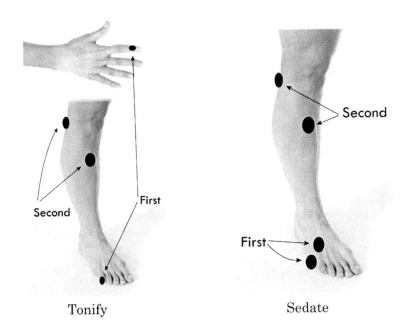

Tonify   Sedate

(e) Bladder meridian

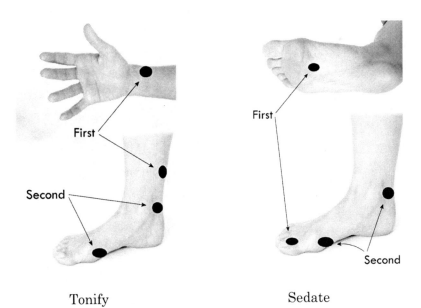

Tonify   Sedate

(f) Kidney meridian

Figure 10.4 *(cont'd)* (g) to (h)

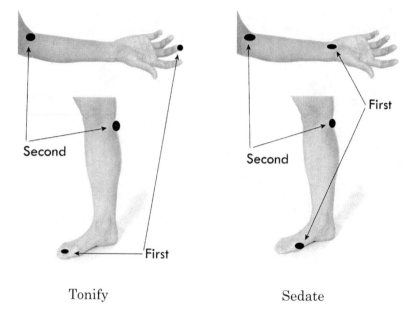

Tonify   Sedate

(g) Circulation-sex meridian

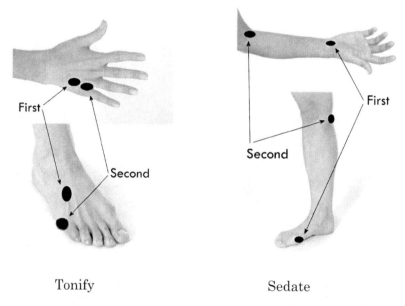

Tonify   Sedate

(h) Triple warmer meridian

Figure 10.4 *(cont'd)* (i) to (j)

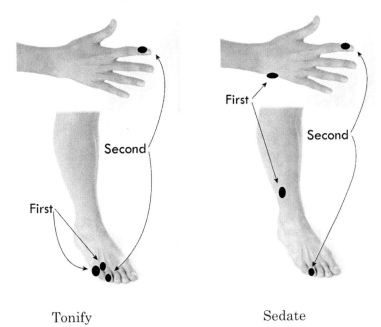

Tonify   Sedate

(i) Gallbladder meridian

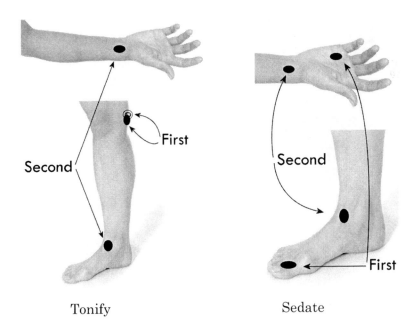

Tonify   Sedate

(j) Liver meridian

Figure 10.4 *(cont'd)* (k) to (l)

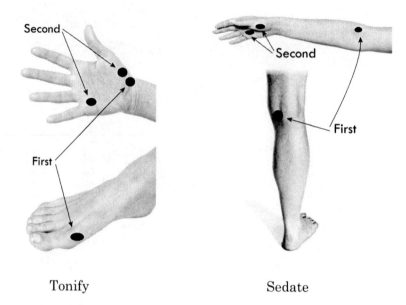

Tonify   Sedate

(k) Liver meridian

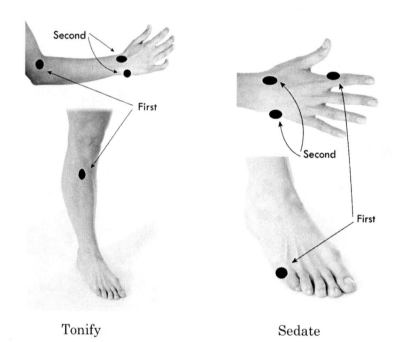

Tonify   Sedate

(l) Large intestine meridian

7   Hold the meridian's acupoints to sedate for 30 seconds or so, or until the pulses under the two pairs of fingers synchronize.

8   Hold the second pair for 20 seconds or so.

9   Recheck the alarm points looking for any remaining over-energy. They should now all be clear.

It is considered much more desirable to tonify under-energized meridians than sedate over-energized ones, and tonifying meridians usually has the effect of balancing over-energized meridians without the need to sedate them.

Warning:

It is recommended that you don't sedate the heart meridian, whether by using acupoints or by tracing the energy flow backwards. (The acupoints that are given in Touch for Health literature to 'sedate' the heart meridian are actually to tonify the small intestine meridian, which has a calming effect on the heart meridian.)

The central and governing meridians form their own inner circuit. If one or both are out of balance, the *central and governing hook up*[1] is a gentle and convenient way of balancing them both.

18 CORRECTION
Central & governing hook up

1   Place the middle finger of one hand gently on the navel and the middle finger of the other between the eyebrows on the forehead.

2   Take a breath and tug upwards slightly with both fingers. Breathe normally.

3   Hold gently for a minute or two or until you can feel the pulses synchronize.

---

1   This comes from Donna Eden, *Energy Medicine* (Piatkus, 1998).

Time of day balance

At any time of day one of the twelve meridians (excluding central and governing) is the most active and has the most influence. Stimulating the meridian that is most active at any particular time helps to balance all the body's energies. To balance your energies and help you feel better right now, give yourself (or someone else) a time of day balance.

The meridian energy wheel (figure 10.5) shows the two-hour time period in which each meridian is most active. To give yourself a time of day balance:

1☐ Trace the meridian associated with the time of day.
2☐ Massage the associated neuro-lymphatic points.
3☐ Hold the associated neuro-vascular points.
4☐ Trace the time-of-day meridian again.

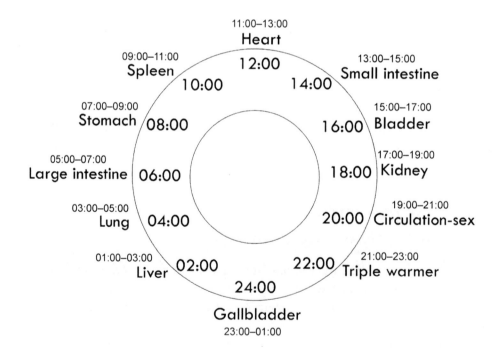

Figure 10.5 The meridian energy wheel

19 CORRECTION
Time of day balance

1 Refer to the meridian wheel (figure 10.5) to find out which meridian is most active right now.
2 Trace this meridian on both sides of the body (one at a time or both at once). (It's particularly nice – but not necessary – if you can get someone to do this for you.)
3 Massage the neuro-lymphatic points related to this meridian.
4 Hold the neuro-vascular points related to this meridian.
5 Trace the meridian again.
6 Optional: check your alarm points (medium pressure). Unless there is something specifically concerning you right now, they will probably all be clear.

A§ **Balancing acupoints**

You recall that, as one of our pre-checks, we trace the central meridian in the direction of energy flow (upwards) and against the flow (downwards). If there is no signal change when we trace the meridian in the direction of energy flow and if there is an signal change when we trace against the flow, we assume that all is well.

However, when we get a signal change after tracing a meridian backwards it means that not all the acupoints are in balance. If all the acupoints were in balance, there would be no signal change when tracing the meridian in either direction. In other words, if every acupoint on a meridian were in balance, the body would have no objection to the meridian being traced the 'wrong' way.

Two eminent kinesiologists, Elizabeth and Hamilton Barhydt, have found that when a meridian is in full balance (i.e. every acupoint on that meridian is in balance), all the muscles associated with that meridian are also in balance.[1] Although we are not specifically addressing muscles in this text, if the Barhydts are right, balancing your acupoints is a very effective way of improving your posture, since you will also be balancing your muscles.

1 Elizabeth Barhydt and Hamilton 'Hap' Barhydt, *Accurate Muscle Testing for Foods and Supplements plus Balancing Meridians*, p. 44.

Take a few minutes to balance the acupoints on one or two of your meridians.
Take your central meridian to start with. The principle is the same for all
the channels. You will ask the pendulum to direct you to the acupoints that
are out of balance; this saves you looking up the location of each acupoint.
The balancing technique will be to hold the point with gentle pressure using
either a positively or negatively charged finger.[1]

20 CORRECTION
Balancing acupoints

1   Trace the meridian in the direction of the energy flow. This should not
produce a signal change. Now trace the meridian backwards (but don't
trace the heart meridian backwards). This would normally produce a
signal change. If the reverse is true, and you get a signal change when
tracing the meridian in the direction of energy flow, there is likely to be
over-energy in the meridian. Correct this by 'flushing': trace the meridian forwards and backwards several times.

2   Let your body know that you're looking for acupoints that are out of
balance. The pendulum will begin to give you an indicator change when
it gets near such an acupoint, but it won't give you the completed,
perpendicular change of swing until you are touching the unbalanced
acupoint in exactly the right place.

3   Starting at the beginning of the meridian, gradually move two fingers
along the channel, in the direction of the energy flow, while holding the
pendulum in your other hand, (For the central meridian, the channel
begins at the perineum and ends just below the middle of your bottom
lip.)

4   When the pendulum begins to swing you know you are near an unbalanced acupoint. Keep moving your two fingers to find exactly the
right spot. You know you have the right spot when the pendulum has
completed the movement of its indicator change and is making the correct swing.

---

1 Adjacent fingers have opposite charges, so the forefinger and the middle finger will have opposite charges. In fact, on the right hand the forefinger is positively charged and the middle finger negatively charged; and on the left hand
this is reversed: the forefinger is negatively charged and the middle finger is
positively charged. (See figure 14.2, page 231.)

5   Now that you have found the point that needs balancing, touch the acupoint with your forefinger alone (using light pressure).

6   If the touch of the forefinger produces an indicator change, hold the finger there. Let your body know you would like an indicator change when the point becomes balanced. Hold the finger there until you get that change. Go to point 8 below.

7   If the touch of the forefinger produces no change, touch the same spot with just your middle finger (using light pressure). This will produce a signal change. Hold this point until a signal change lets you know that the point is now in balance.

8   Going slowly, trace further along the meridian, until the pendulum again begins to change its swing (which won't happen if all the remaining acupoints are in balance). Again, determine the exact spot; find out which finger will balance the point; hold it until you get an indicator change.

9   Continue until the points have all been balanced along the whole length of the meridian.

10   Now trace the meridian in the direction of the flow; and then trace it in the opposite direction. There should be no signal change, even when tracing against the flow of energy. You have successfully balanced all the acupoints on the meridian.

Clearly this method takes time and balancing all the acupoints for all the meridians would be extremely time consuming and impractical. In the context of a goal balance (see part III), it is likely that no more than one specific meridian will require bringing into full balance – just hope it's not the bladder meridian! Even then, you might only need to find one or two priority acupoints to balance the whole meridian; or correcting one or two points might be all your body needs (or can achieve) at that time. Working with priority meridians and priority acupoints will drastically reduce the number of corrections you'll need to make.

Balancing the acupoints on some of your meridians might be tricky. For example, if you are right handed, how do you find the unbalanced acupoints on your left arm (assuming you are holding the pendulum in your right hand)? You need some ingenuity. The following exercise is for balancing the lung meridian, which flows from just below the shoulder to the tip of the thumb.

Exercise 10.2 Balancing the lung meridian

1   Trace the meridian in the direction of the energy flow from below the clavicle near the shoulder to the edge of the thumb nail.

2   Pick up your pendulum, get it swinging on the YES axis, and ask it to respond to the tracing of the channel you have just made. There should be no signal change, since you are encouraging the natural energy flow.

3   Trace the meridian in the other direction, against the natural flow, from thumb to shoulder. Again pick up the pendulum, swing it on the YES axis and ask for a response. If some of the acupoints are out of balance (which is almost certainly the case) you will get an indicator change. Even easier, you could simply ask: *Are there any unbalanced acupoints on the lung meridian?*

4   Now find the individual points which are out of balance. Ask the pendulum to indicate unbalanced acupoints by giving a signal change when you *look* at the specific unbalanced point. This requires concentration.

5   So trace the meridian slowly with your eyes. The pendulum will begin to give a signal change when you are in the right area, and will complete that signal change when you are looking in precisely the right spot.

6   Now imagine placing your forefinger on the spot where you are looking. If you get a signal change, put the pendulum down and hold that spot with your forefinger using gentle pressure for 30 seconds or so.

7   If your imagined forefinger on the spot doesn't produce a signal change, imagine placing your middle finger on the point. You should now get a signal change. Put down the pendulum and hold your middle finger on the spot using gentle pressure for 30 seconds or so.

8   Pick up the pendulum and look at the spot. Now there will be no signal change.

9   Find the next point that produces a signal change by using your eyes, as before, and correct using the same procedure.

10   When all of the indicating points have been corrected, trace the meridian against the natural flow. There will be no signal change, showing that all the points on that meridian are in balance.   A§

Now that you have put your central and lung meridians into full balance, you might want to see how long it lasts. Check them again in a few hours (by tracing backwards). When they go out of balance, you might want to find out what put them out of balance. Use your intuition and ask the pendulum. If appropriate, resolve that issue.

A§ Tracing a meridian against the natural flow

Flushing a meridian (tracing it forwards and backwards a number of times) is a good way of clearing it energetically. And, if you are in pain, it can be useful to run the implicated meridian backwards to ease the over-energy associated with the pain. (But don't run the heart meridian backwards.)

21 CORRECTION
Tracing a meridian backwards to alleviate pain

1   Making the pain site as comfortable as possible, check and correct all the alarm points, till they are all clear.
2   Move your body in such a way that the pain is activated.
3   Evaluate the level of pain or discomfort.
4   Check your alarm points again, using a *light touch*. You are checking for over-energy. If there is more than one implicated meridian, find the priority.
5   Trace the meridian backwards (*not if it's the heart*). You may need to trace it backwards several times. (If it feels more comfortable to flush the meridian, do so.)
6   Check the alarm points again for over-energy. If any more indicate, trace the meridian backwards (or flush it).
7   Re-evaluate the level of pain or discomfort.   A§

Using the corrections

You may want to wait just a little longer before putting these powerful tools into operation together as part of a balance. In chapter 13 you'll learn an overall framework and protocol for working with the therapist within. But if you can't wait that long, good! Follow the instructions in exercise 10.3, using table 10.1 (page 178) for page numbers.

		TEST	CORRECTION
# 1	Auditory perception	66	66
# 2	Visual perception	68	69
# 3	Brain integration (cross-crawl)	78	78
# 4	Brain integration (cross-crawl) with eye movements	–	81
# 5	Tracing the lemniscate for vision	–	82
# 6	Tracing the lemniscate for writing	–	84
# 7	Gait reflexes	84	85
# 8	Emotional stress release (ESR)	91	91
# 9	Frontal–occipital holding	–	98
# 10	Emotional distress release (EDR)	–	99
# 11	Colour balance	–	101
# 12	Acknowledging the involved emotion	–	126
# 13	Identifying the antecedents of an issue	–	131
# 14a	Neuro-lymphatic (NL) reflexes (elements)	154	157
# 14b	Neuro-lymphatic (NL) reflexes (alarm points)	158	157
# 15	Neuro-vascular (NV) reflexes	161	161
# 16	Tracing the meridian (alarm points)	–	163
# 17	Acupoints to tonify and sedate	–	164
# 18	Central & governing hook up	–	171
# 19	Time of day balance	–	173
# 20	Balancing acupoints	–	174
# 21	Tracing a meridian backwards to alleviate pain	–	177

Table 10.1 Corrections

Exercise 10.3 Working with an issue

1   State your problem or goal. A signal change will register it. Take a SUD reading of the problem.
2   Find out which corrections will help. Using the pendulum, say (or point to) the correction (table 10.1). You can take several corrections at a time and, if the pendulum indicates, narrow down to the required corrections. If more than one correction is indicated, find the priority.

Alternatively, apply priority mode while going through the corrections and only one (the priority) should be indicated.

3   After doing the correction, ask whether other corrections are required and refer again to the list.

4   Once you have made the corrections, state the problem or goal again. If there is no signal change it means you have done all you can do for now.

5   Recheck the SUD reading. It will probably have significantly improved.

11
What's the Problem?

Identifying the issues

You are probably working with this book because you have specific issues that you want to address. Indeed, everyone has issues. Even the most healthy and well-adjusted people with loving, stable parents and a happy childhood have issues. Those who claim not to have issues have a very limited sense of self-awareness or are living a notably unchallenging existence. It's not that you will get to a stage where you don't have issues. The idea is that they shouldn't be the *same* issues! A challenging life will present you with new issues. Resolve them as you go along, and you won't continually have to face (or try to bury) the old issues.

All issues are resolvable[1] and all issues that aren't resolved keep coming back until we address them successfully. Too often, people never address them and try to evade them, run away from them, hide from them – often because once upon a time they tried and failed to resolve the issue; or, just as likely, have been prevented by fear from even trying and just hope the problem will go away if they ignore it. Problems don't go away by ignoring or suppressing them; they lay deep roots and exert more authority and control over feelings and behaviour. However, it's never too late to address an issue, however long it's been there or however deeply embedded it is. What becomes more difficult with time is conceiving of living *without* the problem.

---

1   An issue is by definition resolvable. The loss of a loved one, for example, may be a tragedy, but it's not in itself an issue. Nor is the natural sadness felt by the bereaved. Facts aren't issues. Natural responses to events are not issues. The inability to grieve; not being able to recover from the shock of a death; remaining angry long after the event; being in the same place years later – these are examples of issues.

But these techniques can help you with that as well. When you begin to make good progress with your lifetime problem, if you find yourself reluctant to continue and frightened of who you will be if you no longer have the problem, treat that as your issue and resolve it before going any further.

Having an *issue* means experiencing at least one of the following:

1☐ You want to do or get something but something's stopping you from doing it or getting it.
2☐ You are doing or feeling something you don't want to do or feel.
3☐ You have a physical symptom or illness that has an emotional basis.

A goal is distinct from an issue (see chapter 12 about formulating goals). However, they are related. An issue requires a goal (even if the goal is latent and unformulated). A goal is not an issue; but any obstacles interfering with the achievement of a goal constitute issues.

Resolving your issues helps you to achieve your goals and progress in your self-development. It can also greatly improve your energy levels. Most problems have unresolved traumas[1] at their source. Unresolved traumas consume energy. Resolving your issues allows this energy to be available for pursuing your real goals.

Occasionally, clarifying and delineating the problem is all that you need to do in order to resolve it. This is true of problems which exist completely in the present and do not relate to past traumas. In any case, to resolve an issue you should first acknowledge and clarify it.

To clarify a problem tune into the feelings associated with it. Then acknowledge the emotion connected with the feelings (see chapter 7). If the problem relates solely to the present, staying with the emotions will help you to clarify them. Trust whatever comes up and follow it through. If the problem results from past trauma you will need to address it with the pendulum and the methods in this book. If the problem relates solely to your present circumstances, take action to change your circumstances. As you do so, you might come up with issues that prevent you from taking this action. Resolve those issues.

---

1   For an explanation of my use of the word *trauma,* see footnote on page 9.

The key question to ask with the pendulum is, *Do I need more information?* The pendulum will help you to make conscious all the information you need. Once you have made conscious all the information, you can then address the issue with the methods your body selects.

Life indexes

You can do an audit of the quality of your life using *life indexes* (table 11.1, page 185). Use the pendulum – or your conscious judgement – to find out which life indexes would be useful to score (but use your *unconscious* to come up with the scores). There is no need to do all of them at once. You may want to plot a selection of them over time, noticing how they change in response to the work you do using this book. Extra rows are provided in the table for you to add any other indexes that would be useful to you.

If 100 per cent is the ultimate ideal and zero per cent is the worst conceivable state, use the pendulum to give yourself scores for each life index that seems relevant to you now. Alternatively, come up with a figure by using your intuition: consider the life index and let your body come up with a number. When you do this, it's important not to think about it; the number will just come up, and is usually the first thing that comes into your head. It's best to do this quickly. Do *not* use your conscious judgement for this exercise (you won't know if you're fooling yourself).

If you're using a pendulum, the procedure for finding the score is the same for each index, and you are probably familiar with it by now. It's usually a good idea to start at 50 per cent and go up or down as necessary (see example A and B on page 184). If any score seems bizarre, check that you have permission to do this, check the central meridian for over-energy, and check for switching. You can also ask your body if there are any other factors affecting the accuracy of the results (then find out what they are). To make the process quicker, you could choose to round the percentage up or down to the nearest ten.

It might be useful to consider what the different scores mean to you. Is below 50 per cent unacceptable? Is above 80 per cent a very good score? If you consider these questions in advance it will help your body to give you scores that make sense to you. Use the pendulum to guide you.

Example A:

1□ You ask: *Is it as high as 50 per cent?* The response is YES.
2□ *Is it as high as 60 per cent?* YES.
3□ *Is it as high as 70 per cent?* NO.
4□ *Is it as high as 65 per cent?* YES.
5□ *As high as 66?* YES.
6□ *As high as 67?* NO. The percentage is therefore 66.

Example B:

1□ You ask: *Is it as high as 50 per cent?* The response is NO.
2□ *Is it as high as 40 per cent?* NO.
3□ *Is it as high as 30 per cent?* YES.
4□ *As high as 35 per cent?* NO.
5□ *As high as 31 per cent?* YES.
6□ *As high as 32 per cent?* NO.
7□ The percentage is therefore 31.

The meanings of the terms in the life indexes are different for different people. What do they mean to you? The more specific your question and the more defined your terms, the more accurate and meaningful the response. For example, what do you understand by *Quality of environment?* Would it be useful to have separate indexes for work environment and home environment? When you say environment do you mean simply physical environment (clutter, comfort, space) or are you including the atmosphere and quality of energy; or do you need separate indexes for these? What are you going to mean by the index, *Spiritual development?* When you measure for *Quality of nutrition*, what's the time frame you have in mind: your diet (i.e. eating regimen) of the last week, the last month, the last year? Of course, the categories *Satisfaction with face* and *Satisfaction with body* refer to your being at ease with how you look, not your judgement of how pretty you are. The life indexes in table 11.1 are in no particular order.

How do the figures provided by your unconscious body compare with those you might have anticipated consciously? You might want to take a moment to consider this. They may be very similar. If they are very different, this points to a lack of congruence between your conscious and unconscious – which isn't at all surprising if you have significant issues to address. Later, after you've addressed some of these issues, you may find this discrepancy has reduced considerably.

It may be that helping one area of your life automatically helps others. Improving one index may automatically help others, since everything relates to everything else.

Life index		Date	Score /100	Date	Score /100	Date	Score /100
1	Physical health						
2	Physical fitness						
3	Overall happiness						
4	Quality of relationship						
5	Quality of sexual life						
6	Self-esteem						
7	Quality of nutrition						
8	Satisfaction with face						
9	Satisfaction with body						
10	Quality of sleep						
11	Spiritual development						
12	Quality of environment						
13	Taking time for self						
14	Satisfaction with work						
15	Emotional health						
16	Living your life mission						
17	Quality of friendships						
18	At peace with self						
19							
20							
21							

Table 11.1 Life indexes

Life choices

Consider the *life choices* in table 11.2 (page 187). Use the pendulum to find out which statements are relevant to you (or the priority) right now (or relevant to your goal or issue). Then find out the extent to which you believe them or their degree of truth using the validity of cognition (VOC) scale.

The VOC scale is a subjective seven-point scale (1 to 7), which measures the strength of a belief. The belief should be in the form of a statement in the first person and in the present tense. For example, *I choose to accept responsibility for my decisions.* (All the statements in table 11.2 are in this format.) Give the statement a score between 1 and 7, where 1 means you hardly believe it at all and 7 means you believe it absolutely.

The VOC scale is a useful supplement to the SUD scale. The SUD measures the quality of the problem; the VOC measures the belief in the goal. You can use the pendulum or your intuition.

22 CORRECTION
Working with life choices

1☐   Identify the priority life choices statements from table 11.2.
2☐   State each priority life choice out loud.
3☐   Give each a VOC score (using your intuition or the pendulum).
4☐   Identify the issues that relate to the statements and address them with the methods learned.

Some of the life choices statements may require a third-person perspective to make sense of them. For example, *I choose to express my emotions appropriately.* It's possible you don't know how or in what circumstances to express an emotion appropriately. If this is the case, talk to a therapist or other disinterested person. Alternatively, model the perspective of a third person yourself.[1]

23 CORRECTION
Modelling a third-person perspective

1☐   Choose a person whose wisdom and perspective you admire. They can be known personally to you or they can be a public figure, a historical figure, or even a fictional character.

---

1 Modelling is a central tool of NLP. Indeed NLP was founded on modelling successful therapists.

1   I choose to be happy.
2   I choose to acknowledge and accept my emotions.
3   I choose to express my emotions appropriately.
4   I choose to accept myself as I am and allow myself to change.
5   I choose to be free.
6   I choose to give myself time.
7   I choose to love, respect and value myself.
8   I choose to accept responsibility for my life.
9   I choose to allow others to take responsibility for themselves.
10 I choose to fulfil my potential.
11 I choose to respect and feel free to disagree with others' judgements.
12 I choose to accept my mortality.
13 I choose to accept the right of others to have opinions of me that I disagree with.
14 I choose to accept, learn from and let go of the past.
15 I choose to be true to myself.
16 I choose to deserve abundance.
17 I choose to let go of self-imposed limitations.
18 I choose to appreciate the positive intentions behind the negative and destructive behaviour of others.
19 I choose to forgive myself.
20 I choose to forgive others.
21 I choose to trust myself.
22 I choose to trust the universe.
23 I choose to trust trustworthy people.
24 I choose to allow myself to make mistakes and learn from them.
25 I choose to allow others to make mistakes.
26 I choose to be confident.
27 I choose emotionally healthy, supportive people to be close to me.
28 I choose a partner who allows me space to be myself and continue to develop freely.
29 I choose to allow my partner space to be him/herself and continue to develop freely.
30 I choose to express my needs and desires appropriately.
31 I choose to assert my opinions appropriately.
32 I choose to express myself fully.
33 I choose to embrace all the possibilities of life.
34 I choose to express my sexuality freely and appropriately.
35 I choose to resolve my issues.
36 I choose to be physically healthy.
37 I choose to be a spiritual being.
38 I choose to love and be loved.

Table 11.2 Life choices

2▢   Select a separate chair for them to sit on or a place for them to stand.
3▢   Occupy that space and imagine you are stepping into that person's body and experience what it's like to be that person, looking through their eyes and hearing with their ears.
4▢   As that person, voice your opinion about whatever it is for which a third-person perspective is required.
5▢   When you have got all the information you need, step out of the person's body, and thank them.
6▢   Step back into your own body and imagine you are applying that person's perspective in whatever situations require it. Use ESR for future performance if it would help (page 93).

Modelling a third person is immensely useful whenever you feel stuck in a way of thinking or being. If you can't do it, or find it very difficult to do, it may be that it would be helpful to improve your powers of observation. Study other people a little more closely. Get out of yourself and enter someone else's world. Notice their movements, gestures, expressions. Try them out and notice how you feel as you do so. Aim to change and develop your own language of behaviour. Do it consciously, at first, and your unconscious body will learn quickly. Doing so may improve your powers of empathy.

Motivation for change

Making the decision to heal and to address significant issues is not an easy one. Following that through to the end, wherever it might lead, can be even more difficult. It may require considerable commitment and motivation. However, it's always worth it; it's usually much easier than you think; and it might be completed very quickly.

Ask yourself this shocking question: *If I keep doing this* [the problem: working too hard, smoking, eating badly, neglecting your own health or interests], *how long should I expect to live?* Allow your intuition – or the pendulum – to come up with an age. Then ask yourself: *If I overcome this and change my behaviour, how long can I expect to live?* (Of course you do not have final control over your destiny and the gods may have other plans for you.) The answers can help motivate change. For most issues the primary benefit is happiness and health, but the consequence could be a longer life.

If I keep this problem/doing this my potential lifespan is	
If I resolve this my potential lifespan becomes	

Table 11.3 Lifespan choice

If ever you are feeling that you are losing motivation, let lack of motivation be your issue, and use the techniques here to improve your motivation and energy to work through your problems.

Perhaps you need some help and support to motivate you to make the changes. The following method, # 24, based on Robert Dilts' *Generative NLP*, allows you to create your own personal cheerleaders.

24 CORRECTION
Generating a support system

1␍ Identify a behaviour or activity for which you'd like to generate support.

2␍ Identify a number of people who you'd like to support you in this behaviour or activity. It doesn't matter whether the people are known to you or not; and they can even be fictional characters. You need at least three people, but you can have as many as you like. It is helpful if one person knew you in the past; a second knows you in the present; and a third is someone who will know you in the future.

3␍ Make sure you have some floor space to work in. The space behind you will be occupied by the persons who knew you in the past; the space to the side of you by the persons who know you in the present; the space in front of you by the persons who will know you in the future.

4␍ Step out of your own body (imaginatively), and take a step backwards into the body of a person from the past. Imagine you are now that person. Give some encouraging words from that person in the past to the you in the present. It might be, for example: *You were such a lively child, full of energy and enthusiasm for life; I know this is still inside you and you can use it to help you be the person you want to be.*

5␍ Step back inside your body, face that person, and imagine hearing his or her words to you.

6␍ Repeat with any other characters from the past.

7□   Step to the side, into the body of a person in the present. Again imagin-
      ing you are that person, give some encouraging words from that person
      in the present. Step back into your own body and hear that person's
      words.
8□   Repeat with any other characters in the present.
9□   Take a step forward and do the same process with the person(s) who
      will know you in the future.

Stressors and energizers

It can be very useful to take a reading of your levels of stress and available
energy related to a current issue. Decide on the issue, and use the pendulum
to determine the percentage of stress and energy. Take a reading of the levels
of stress and energy before you address any issue, and again after you have
worked on the issue.

Stressors are anything your body doesn't have adequate resources to deal
with comfortably. You might think of a horse pulling a load that's too heavy
for it. It will manage for a while, but pull the load for too long (or encounter
a very steep hill) and the beast will become exhausted. If such demands are
sustained over a period, the animal will suffer ill health. Identifying and
either eliminating or resolving some of your stressors is a very effective way
of improving the quality of your life.

Issue	% Stress	% Energy

Table 11.4 Levels of stress and available energy related to a current issue

Whether your symptoms are problems with your skin, digestion, or lack of
self-confidence, there may be a number of stressors that your body is trying
to cope with. Stress is cumulative. There is a threshold beyond which your
body ceases to work efficiently because too much energy is engaged in trying

to cope with the stressors. Compare this to the horse pulling a load. If the load is light enough and the horse is powerful enough, there's no problem. But if the metaphorical load is too heavy, you either have too many small stressors to carry, or the few stressors are particularly weighty. The stressors may be relatively new; or they may have been with you a long time and seem a part of you.

If your body is besieged by overwork, insufficient relaxation, poor nutrition, pollutants in the environment, and unresolved emotional traumas, it's not surprising if it is not coping well. What *appears* as the problem might only be the final straw. The real problem is not the final straw but the cumulation of stressors. Your aim is to get the load (your stressors) below the critical level. When this happens, many previous stressors will no longer pose a challenge to your system.

Similarly, identifying your *energizers* will help you to combat the ill effects of the stressors you are subject to. Your energizers are those activities and experiences which support you, strengthen you, and improve the quality of your life. Like a see-saw, the greater the weight of your energizers with respect to your stressors, the better able you are to cope with the stressors. Boosting your energizers is equivalent to giving more power to the horse. The stronger the horse, the greater load it can carry. Stressors which are not major or significant will have a disproportionately detrimental effect if you aren't doing some of the things that support and revivify you.

Using the see-saw as a pair of scales, you can weigh up each side and make sure that your energizers are greater than your stressors. Most people need to increase their energizers; people spend too much time working and not enough pursuing their interests and enjoying their relationships. But even if your energizers are significantly greater than your stressors, it is still very important to resolve your stressors. By doing so, you promote your health and happiness.

Caroline Myss, when considering people with serious and potentially terminal illnesses, makes a helpful distinction between *the desire to live* and *the desire to heal*. Just about everyone wants to live, she asserts, but far fewer are prepared to heal.[1] By concentrating solely on your energizers, you are demonstrating that desire to live; by resolving your stressors you are demon-

---

1   Caroline Myss & C. Norman Shealy, *The Creation of Health* (Bantam Books, Reading, UK).

strating your commitment to *heal*. Similarly, everyone wants to be healthy, but far fewer people are prepared to *change*. *Healing often requires change.* Changing involves consciousness, will and courage.

Take a few minutes to consider your stressors and energizers (table 11.5). Again, you can use the pendulum or your intuition. You'll be using a scale from +10 (greatest source of energy) to −10 (highest level of stress). For each issue: (1) Determine a minus score (−1 to −10) for your stressors; (2) determine a plus score for your energizers (+1 to +10). Again, you can plot changes of score over time as you address your chosen issues; or you can address these areas directly.

Most of the categories in the table are self-evident and should be interpreted in any way most helpful to you. The category *diet* refers to all the foods you eat, which may include foods you are sensitive or allergic to and includes the stress to your metabolic system, as well as the pleasure (or guilt), of eating your favourite foods. Each category may refer not only to the present but to unresolved issues from the past. For example, you might have a very good relationship with your current partner, but there are stressors from the past that are sometimes triggered in your present relationship. Or things might now be fine in relation to your parents, but further inside you are harbouring unresolved anger and resentment because of how things were when you were a child.

Remember this: unresolved problems remain a drain on your resources; but *a difficult experience or relationship, once resolved, becomes a resource.* It's from the difficulties and mistakes that you learn most. But it's your choice. You can choose not to learn from the difficult times. You can choose to be a victim. Or you choose to regard such challenges positively. No one but you will benefit if you do the latter.

You will probably register a stress score in each category. It is the human condition that circumstances and events – sometimes even those that are the most fulfilling – cause stress. You have no control over that. But you can choose to resolve the causes of unnecessary stress and you can choose to engage in energizing activities. For the *mean* (mean average) column, add your stress and energy together. For example, if you stress at work (tasks) is −4 and your energy from work is +8, you get a mean score of +4. Take a separate pendulum reading for your *overall* stress and energy at the bottom of the table.

	Date	Stress −SUD	Energy +SUD	Mean	Date	Stress −SUD	Energy +SUD	Mean	Date	Stress −SUD	Energy +SUD	Mean
Diet/nutrition (incl. allergies & sensitivities)												
Emotional life												
Family												
Friendships												
Hopes and dreams												
Leisure interests												
Other activities												
Physical environment												
Physical exercise												
Relationship with partner												
Relationships at work												
Work (tasks)												
Other												
OVERALL												

Table 11.5 Stressors and energizers

Health–happiness indicators

Finally, the health–happiness indicators are a very useful way of measuring your overall health and state of being. Give each a score relating to how you are in the present (over the last 10 days or so – determine a time frame that suits you), where zero is the worst conceivable state and ten the best you could possibly experience. For this exercise use your *conscious mind* to come up with the figures; it concerns your conscious experience as an expression of your current stress/energizer levels. As you apply the techniques in this text to your issues, very soon you will find the scores going up.

1   Comfort in body

Date					
Score / 10					

This refers to the surface of your body (skin, orifices and so on) as well as the interior (muscles, organs and so on). How relaxed is your body in normal, everyday life? How comfortable does your body feel? Awareness of your somatic experience gives you awareness of the messages your unconscious body is communicating and the possibility of responding. However, these communications can be very uncomfortable. Generally, the more uncomfortable they are, the more imperative the message. Be aware of tension in muscles and compensations (as certain muscles do the job of other muscles), as well as aches, strains and pains in any part of the body. Tension in your muscles means you're holding on to something. Don't ignore your symptoms! Use your pendulum to find out more about them and what you can do to remedy them.

2   Quality of sleep

Date					
Score / 10					

This involves: (1) going to bed at a reasonable time; (2) ease in falling asleep; (3) sleeping soundly through the night; (4) having sufficient sleep; (5) waking refreshed; and (6) general wakefulness during the day.

3 Ease of eating/digesting

Date					
Score / 10					

How does your body, and specifically your stomach feel after eating? Are you tired after a meal? Does your body react to any of the foods you eat (with itchiness of the skin or spots, bloating, stomach ache and so on)? Is your digestive system working properly? Are your bowel movements regular (once or twice a day), or do you get constipated, or suffer from loose bowels?

4 Appropriateness of moods

Date					
Score / 10					

The important thing is that your moods are appropriate to your experience. A score of 10/10 indicates experiencing entirely *appropriate* moods, not necessarily elation or joy. Moods should not be extreme or prolonged without good cause. Do you have frequent unexplained mood swings? It is important to be able to feel and express appropriately the full range of emotions – including, for example, anger, fear, sadness, joy, gratefulness, longing. If you think you have a problem acknowledging or expressing emotions, use your pendulum and the five-element emotion chart (on page 124) to find which emotion presents a problem and what the problem is. This tends to be a particular problem for men, since men are discouraged from acknowledging feelings of hurt or vulnerability and are encouraged to express hurt through aggression. Women, however, often find it difficult to cope with their own or others' feelings of aggression and suppress or disavow such feelings or express them vicariously. The suppression of feelings is also standard among people who smoke or take other legal or illegal drugs to chemically mask their feelings.

5   Level of concentration and motivation

Date					
Score / 10					

This may include your motivation to get up in the morning, to get a task or a job done, to pursue an interest, or to get ahead with your career. You may have difficulty concentrating on your work, or on the task at hand. The problem might be specific to one area, or generalized over many. Again, the pendulum can help you to identify the problem and rectify it.

Introjecting others' problems

When considering the genesis of your problems there is a possibility that the problem isn't yours at all. It is not at all uncommon that people introject their parents' problems and carry them as if they were their own. If you are having difficulty identifying the source of your problem, consider the possibility that it is your father or mother's problem (usually but not always the mother).

Parental problems often take a physical form when introjected, such as pain or discomfort in the throat or abdomen. They manifest in behaviour that is not fully understood – for good reason, since the behaviour is either what the parent wants, or is a compensation. The consequence of this is that such a person doesn't know who he or she is, because a significant part of the person is a quality of the parent.

Examples of introjection of parental issues include fear or pain regarding sex, rejection, self-expression, separation. But the introjected parental problem can be anything, including (commonly) the need to parent the parents, or putting on a happy face and pretending that nothing's wrong.

If you suspect that your problem may belong to one (or both) of your parents, ask the pendulum about it. Get as much information as you can. You might not get it all at once! Allow processing time.[1] If necessary, consider contacting a good therapist.

As well as using kinesiology methods you can symbolically return the problem to your parent. The following exercise is inspired by an exercise devised by Robert Dilts.[2]

25 CORRECTION
Giving the problem back (1)

1☐ Identify a problem that belongs to one or both of your parents. (If the problem comes from someone who isn't your parent, replace parent with this person throughout the exercise.)

2☐ Get in touch with the feelings related to the problem. Notice where you feel it in your body.

3☐ Become aware that this is not your stuff; it is alien to you.

4☐ Let those alien feelings constitute a substance, and let your body tell you what that substance would be. (It might be weeds, branches, threads, or a deposit of some sort, for example.) Become aware of this substance inside you. Notice the texture and smell of this substance.

5☐ Take the substance out of your body. It may need to come from your stomach, throat, head, or some other part of you. Do this as if physically. Use your hands to help you. Keep going until you have removed every shred, strand or grain of it.

6☐ Present this mass of substance back to your parent(s) (in your imagination of course, since they probably have nowhere to put it); or dispose of it in whatever way you choose (again, entirely in your imagination: you might choose to burn it or bury it in land or at sea, or even rocket it into space).

7☐ Notice how you feel now. You might sense a lightness and relief. You might also be aware of something missing.

---

1 Processing time is the time your unconscious body needs between self-kinesiology sessions to work through the changes you have instigated. This processing time requires no efforts on the part of your conscious mind; it works completely automatically.

2 In *Tools of the Spirit*, by Robert Dilts and Robert McDonald (Meta Publications, 1997). Also see Giving the problem back (2), # 34, page 249.

8☐   Imagine yourself as more of how you would like to be: confident, relaxed, happy, and totally yourself. The imaginary you is a little further than you are right now in spiritual evolution. But make sure this imaginary you is *not* perfect, nor an ideal you, but has a sense of humour. Let a picture form of this new self form.

9☐   Make sure the more evolved you is appealing. See this you in three dimensions.

10☐   Open your arms and accept this new you – who is actually the real you, the you who you would always have been if you hadn't been carrying your parents' issues – into your body. If there was a part of you where you felt something was missing, bring the new you into there.

11☐   Allow this new you to integrate.

12
What Do You Want?

Your focus might be on the problem, or it might be on the goal. The former is often referred to as therapy; the latter coaching. But any problem has an implicit goal, just as any goal which requires assistance has an implicit problem. The dual elements of problem and goal are implicit in any issue. The most effective coaching encompasses therapy, and vice-versa.

It's important to resolve the problem, but your *focus* should be on what you want, not on what you're trying to get away from. If you focus on the problem, it's likely to stay with you. If you keep your eye on something, you should expect to keep seeing it. Direct your attention on to what you want and your energies will direct you towards it.

It's also *motivating* to focus on the goal. If, for example, you think about all the effort involved in doing a project, it can easily lose its appeal. But if you focus on the achievement and consider how wonderful it will be to have completed the project, you will be motivated to get on with it.

You have conscious control over your thoughts and your will. Use your consciousness to think positively and act purposefully.

Before determining the exact wording of your goal, make sure you have permission to work with the general goal. Also ask the pendulum if this is the most appropriate goal to be working with right now. If it isn't, you might want to find out what is. If you do have permission and it is the appropriate goal to be working with, the next step is to establish the precise wording of your goal: the goal statement.

Any goal should have the following features:

1☐ It is described in positive terms.
2☐ It is under your own control.
3☐ It is realistic, achievable and worthwhile.

1 The goal is described in positive terms

This is worth reiterating. The goal is what you want, not what you don't want; it is an affirmation, not a negation. By focusing on the goal, you give yourself a positive outcome to aim for, rather than something to avoid. For example, if you're concerned not to feel anxious, you're preoccupied with the exact thing you want to avoid – which makes you more likely to feel anxious. (Try not thinking about a pink elephant wearing a yellow scarf!)[1]

If your problem is nervousness or anxiety when speaking in front of a group, ask yourself what you want instead of nervousness and anxiety. You might determine to be confident and relaxed. Your goal would then be: *I am confident and relaxed when speaking in front of a group.*

2 The goal is under your own control

This is about boundaries and self-responsibility. Make sure that your goal is to help your own responses and behaviour, not somebody else's.

If the goal is *not* under your control – if, for example, it is about changing the behaviour of someone else – it is an inappropriate goal. You can't change the behaviour of someone else; you can't *make* anyone change. In fact, you may well be able to facilitate change in your partner, but not by choosing that as your goal. Your partner may well change as an indirect consequence of you changing. You have no right to demand that another person changes if it is against their will. It is always their choice. You can *encourage* others to change. You can *sponsor* them as they change themselves. You can even *ask* someone to make changes. But you can't make anyone change. It's pointless to demand that someone changes. You don't have that power (moral, or phys-

---

1 This is how parents and educators get it wrong when they tell those in their care what *not* to do. By pointing out what they shouldn't be doing, they're very likely to do it – not through malice but because that is what their attention is focused on.

ical) – unless, perhaps, you have a private army. It is hard enough to change oneself! Trying to change somebody else is one of the greatest stresses in life and invariably a mistake. The challenge is to accept yourself and others, and do what you can to develop yourself. However, you can change your own inappropriate responses; and you can change your circumstances.

If someone's behaviour is inoffensive but simply bugs you, it's your problem, not theirs. They may be willing to change if you ask (especially if you acknowledge that it's your problem); or you can change your response. The pendulum can help you do this. Acknowledge your response, take responsibility for it, and work on it. This is the key to successful professional, personal and intimate relationships.

However, if your partner's behaviour is unacceptable to you and he or she is unwilling to change, you may want to consider ending the relationship. If you've had uncaring or abusive partners in the past, your goal might be to choose a partner who is kind, warm and able to communicate. These are choices under your control. Better still, resolve that thing in yourself that attracts you to unsuitable partners. Then your present relationship will probably naturally come to an end and you will pick more suitable partners in the future. Addressing the cause rather than the symptom of the problem takes courage and effort, but it is the most effective course.

It may seem that what stops you achieving your goal (for example, of having a successful relationship or a satisfying job) is something outside of your control. For example, your partner invariably turns out to be untrustworthy or abusive; or whatever job you get your boss puts you down. But in all probability there is something in you that perpetuates this situation. If you keep encountering or repeating the same problem, it is more than simply bad luck! The unconscious body will keep presenting the issue until you address it and resolve it. This is actually positive and useful. As you have already read in these pages, all issues are *opportunities* to resolve something in yourself, usually deriving from the past, promoting self-development.

The issue of self-responsibility and boundaries is involved in the majority of clients who present themselves for therapy. It has fundamentally two manifestations:

1☐ *Assuming responsibility for others*
   Other people's problems become your problem. You restrict your behaviour, desires, words to save another from – you think – feeling

bad, even when your desired behaviour would bring you happiness and would not bring any detriment to the other person.

2☐ *Living other people's agendas (and allowing others to be responsible for you)*

If you do this, your behaviour, your desires, even your values, are not your own. Instead of choosing these things for yourself you let others choose for you. You may be living your parents' agenda and values; those of your boss or work colleagues; or those of any influential people in your life.

To illustrate point 1: Amanda; (not her real name) was reluctant to be successful in her work and even have children because she feared her sister would be jealous and resentful. Amanda was unclear of her boundaries and was not clear about where she stopped and her sister began. She took responsibility for her sister's feelings and tried to protect her from behaviour that might upset her. This didn't help her sister or herself. If this truly was an issue for her sister (rather than just Amanda's own projections), then it was something for her sister to address, rather than be protected from. And if Amanda sacrifices herself for her sister, she will end up resenting her. She may not want to acknowledge that resentment (which, after all, wasn't her sister's fault, but her own choice) and her suppressed anger will find expression in unpredictable and insidious ways.

To illustrate point 2: Sasha (not her real name) had been receiving IVF treatment but had still been unable to get pregnant. Her friends were getting pregnant and having children, and Sasha felt under pressure to do the same. However, when she acknowledged her feelings she realized that what she really wanted to do was run away. The truth was that she wasn't ready to have a baby. Her father had died a number of years before and, since his death, in loyalty to him she'd been living according to his agenda rather than her own. She realized that if she had a child she would then have to live according to the agenda of her child, never having the opportunity to be who she wanted. Within a couple of months of this acknowledgement, Sasha was pregnant without medical interference.

This route (of sacrificing interests) may superficially seem the morally good one, but it leads to emotional contortions as true feelings are disallowed. Eventually, the self-sacrificing person becomes a martyr: their life is sacrificed for the benefit of others – who will never appreciate their sacrifices anyway. The martyr is convinced that the sacrifice is made for others but it is really for the martyr's own sake. The martyr, by the way, always harbours resentments, however hidden or denied.

If you tend to take responsibility for others, you can begin to define your issue and address it using the techniques given here. Set yourself goals to work on, such as *I deserve to do what's best for me*; or *I look after my own interests first.*

You may like to consider this as a guiding principle: *what is truly in your own best interests is also in the best interests of others.* Exploiting or deliberately hurting other people cannot be in anyone's best interests. Nor is it in others' best interests to dishonestly 'protect' them from hurt (by, for example, pretending you still love them when you don't). Looking after yourself and making a positive impact on the world are mutually compatible enterprises. Sacrificing yourself for another is rarely in anybody's best interests. Of course it is good to help, support and sponsor others. But not to the detriment of yourself. And, obviously, unless you're looking after yourself you're not going to be much benefit to anyone else. Isn't this the case?

If you tend to live according to other people's agendas, it may be that you don't have a strong sense of self. You may not know what you want or what your own values are; or you may feel guilty about something from the past. You probably don't have much faith in your own judgement – or perhaps you don't even know what your own judgement is. Becoming and honouring yourself may take a little time. Even for relatively healthy people who have a clear sense of self, being true to yourself and becoming who you are is a lifelong challenge.

But if you work through your issues by setting yourself appropriate goals, you will gradually delineate your boundaries, develop your own sense of self, and learn to trust in your own judgement – while being patient and tolerant with yourself (and others).[1]

So let go of the desire to change others. If you have difficulty doing this, address this issue by formulating an appropriate goal.

To take responsibility for your goal you need to *own* it. Use the first person pronoun *I*.

---

1   Intolerance of others is always, at heart, an intolerance of oneself. All malice directed externally is a projection of what's going on inside.

3 The goal is realistic and achievable

Having long-term, very ambitious goals is highly commendable and perfectly reasonable. But these goals mustn't be pie in the sky. Do you believe your goals are possible? If not, is this because the goal is truly unrealistic; or is it because you don't believe in yourself enough?

If the goal is unrealistic, change the goal. Make it something that is within your grasp – but grasp the stars and the heavens.

If you don't believe in yourself enough, then let it be your goal to believe in your own abilities and talents. The following statements[1] often help in finding the cause or nature of a problem; they may lead you to what is preventing you from achieving your goal.

> 1☐ I deserve to have this goal.
> 2☐ I am capable of achieving this goal.
> 3☐ It's possible for me to achieve this goal.
> 4☐ I take responsibility for achieving this goal.
> 5☐ This goal is worth my commitment and effort.

Rather than a yes-or-no answer, it's more meaningful to find out how much you believe the statements. Use the seven-point VOC scale (where one represents *Hardly believe it at all* and seven represents *Believe it absolutely*), and give each statement a score between one and seven.

Even if your goal is realistic and achievable, do you know what you have to do to achieve it? Sometimes a long-term and broadly defined goal needs to be broken down into more specific, shorter term goals. You need to know the route to achieving the broader goal; you need to know the steps that will get you there. The shorter term goals give you signposts on the way. So ask your pendulum if your goal is specific enough. By making your goal specific, and by imagining yourself doing it, you are helping to direct your unconscious body to attain it.

It is also most effective to use the *present tense*, and to state your goal as if it were happening right now, in the present. For example, *I deserve a loving partner*; *I am open and confident when criticized*; *I am assertive with my manager*. If you can't put your goal in the present tense, or when you do so

---

1   Adapted from the work of Robert Dilts, an NLP pioneer (master practitioner materials, 2001).

the goal does not make sense, you have formulated the wrong goal (see the next section).

To recap:

- ○   Check that you have permission to work with the goal.
- ○   State the goal in positive terms, concentrating on what you want.
- ○   Ensure the goal is realistic and achievable (but reach for the stars).
- ○   State the goal in the first person.
- ○   Use the present tense.

Making the goal specific

Initially, your conception of your goal might be the attainment of a particular outcome, which may not be under your direct control. The idea is to make this more specific so that it becomes something you are in control of. This specific goal will enable you to identify the issues that are holding you back.

Imagine, for example, that your outcome is to gain promotion at work.

Goal → *To gain promotion at work.*

Of course you can't guarantee you'll get the promotion. That's in the hands of the gods (and sometimes those who think they are). What you can do is give yourself the best possible chance. You can do this by making sure you put in place everything *that you are responsible for* so that you are thoroughly prepared.

Your goal statement should be in the first person and in the present tense. Conforming to these rules, this (provisional) goal statement would read: *I am promoted at work*. Not only is that not something in your control, it doesn't make sense, since however prepared you are you are not promoted! Putting your goal statement into this format (first person, present tense) is a way of testing that you have the right goal statement. *Your optimum goal statement won't be true in the present (or it wouldn't be a goal), but there has to be the possibility of it being true.*

Goal → *To be thoroughly prepared.*

Provisional goal statement: *I am thoroughly prepared.*

This is a better goal statement. It has the possibility of being true. But it can be broken down even further. How will you know if you are thoroughly prepared? What does being thoroughly prepared involve? To be thoroughly prepared in this instance you have to make sure that you have all the *qualities* and *characteristics* required for your outcome. These are under your control and will give you the best chance of achieving promotion. You might identify, for example, that greater assertiveness and more self-assurance are what you need to help you to be thoroughly prepared.

> Goal → *Greater assertiveness and more self-assurance in all aspects of work.*

> Provisional goal statement: *I am assertive and self-assured in all aspects of my work.*

Is this how you need to be to give you the best chance of promotion? If so, this will be your goal statement.

> Goal statement → *I am assertive and self-assured in all aspects of my work.*[1]

You might equally have ended up with an alternative goal such as *I have all the self-confidence I need to achieve promotion*; *I deserve to be wealthy and content*; or *I am prepared to exercise responsible power over others.*

The goal you end up with will link directly with your issues and bring them into sharp relief.

The most effective goal is as specific and accurate as possible. You can use the pendulum to make sure that you have the best wording for the goal (see exercise 12.1). Choosing the optimum wording for your goal is just about as important as the work you do on it. Expending efforts on a goal that isn't well formulated is uneconomic and is likely to lead to confusion. Defining the goal precisely isn't just a prerequisite for the work you do, it is an essential part of the work itself.

---

1   Even this goal could be more specific. Use the pendulum to ask your body if this goal is specific enough. Ask yourself: How would I know if I were more assertive? What would I be doing that's different? The answer might be, *I am calm and positive when questioned or challenged.* This would then be your goal. There may be a number of goals to work on under the issue of being assertive and self-assured.

Always write down your goal. The precise wording is important, and you will need to repeat it word for word at the conclusion of the balance.

By formulating the goal you are, at the same time, unconsciously determining and tuning in to the problem and what has contributed to it.

Exercise 12.1 Ascertaining the optimum wording for the goal

1   Use the pendulum to check whether the goal you have in mind is, in general terms, the right one: *Is this the right goal to be working with right now?* If not, find the goal you should be working with.
2   Ask: *Have I got exactly the right wording?* If you have the exact wording, you can begin to work on the issue.
3   If you do not have exactly the right wording, ask: *Do I need to add anything?* If so, find out what and add it.
4   Ask: *Do I need to take anything away?* If so find out what and take it away.
5   Keep going until you have precisely the right wording. Your intuition will help you if you give it a chance.

Up to this point you have been addressing individual issues in isolation with the methods you have learned. In kinesiology the methods are usually used in the context of a *balance*. You are now ready to give yourself a balance working with a goal (exercise 12.2). In the next chapter a protocol for self-kinesiology will be outlined so that you can give yourself a full balance. In part III you will learn more techniques to add to your repertoire and apply to your issues.

Exercise 12.2 Balancing with a goal

1   Determine a goal and ask permission from your body to work with it.
2   Formulate the optimum wording and check it with the pendulum.
3   Write down your goal and take a VOC reading.
4   Imagine that you are performing your goal, or doing what you need to do in order to achieve it. Notice the feelings that interfere. The good feelings are helpful, but ignore them for now. Focus on the uncomfortable feelings that interfere with achieving this goal. If these feelings aren't immediately apparent, stay with it until you're in touch with

them. You're looking for somatic feelings in your abdomen or chest (thorax).

5   Get in touch with these somatic feelings.
6   Tune in to the feelings and acknowledge the emotion. Take a SUD reading.
7   Apply the techniques presented so far.
8   Again imagine performing the goal.
9   Recheck the SUD and VOC scores.
10   Thank your body for its help.

13
The Balance

Balancing your energies in relation to a goal means balancing all aspects of your being, since energy incorporates everything. The full balance is similar to what you might experience working with a kinesiologist, except that you will be using a pendulum instead of muscle testing.

The self-kinesiology balance will give you some or all of the following benefits. It will help to:

1 ☐ Clarify your goal.
2 ☐ Make your goal easier to achieve.
3 ☐ Resolve issues arising from the past.
4 ☐ Remove bad feelings.
5 ☐ Transform outdated beliefs.
6 ☐ Improve your physical health.
7 ☐ Give you a sense of happiness, freedom and peace.

You won't always have time to give yourself a full balance. The mini-balance can be accomplished within minutes and allows you to work with a specific problem in the present rather than formulating a goal and resolving the past issues that have contributed to it.

A§ The mini-balance using *circuit lock*[1]

Circuit lock is a way of locking information (such as a problem) in the body in such a way as to make it available and online (described as being 'in circuit').

---

1 *Circuit lock* is also called *pause lock* and *circuit retaining mode* in kinesiology.

When a problem is put into circuit lock every correction you make will be in relation to that problem until the circuit lock is terminated.

If, for example, a particular problem is playing up and you don't have time to do a full balance, simply take the problem into circuit, using circuit lock. All responses from the pendulum will then be in relation to the problem in circuit, allowing you to find the most effective instant remedy.

To put a piece of information into circuit lock:

1□ Bring both feet together (in order to terminate anything that was already in circuit lock, even if only accidentally) and then put the feet at least 18 inches apart to open your legs.[2] Any information is then stored online in your system, ready to be acted upon.[3] Or:

2□ Stroke upwards once or twice, reasonably firmly, with two fingers or the thumb, from the glabella (midway between the eyebrows) to the hairline.

To terminate a circuit, bring the legs together or tap the brow.

Using muscle testing, a kinesiologist will put information into circuit as the muscle is tested. For example, the client will think about a specific situation as the kinesiologist tests an indicator muscle. If the situation causes stress, the muscle unlocks. As the muscle unlocks the legs are put together and immediately apart or the brow is stroked firmly upwards.[4]

With a pendulum you will work in a similar way. Introduce information (for example, a specific situation in your past) or a stimulus (such as a food substance). As the pendulum registers a signal change – i.e. *while* it is changing its swing – take the information into circuit either by putting your legs apart or by stroking upwards on your brow.

---

2   If you are seated, put the knees wide apart to open the legs. It's as if the body is sending information to the brain warning that you are in a vulnerable position and, in addition to this information, any other information at the time of opening the legs is simultaneously registered.

3   If for any reason you are unable to put your legs apart, open your mouth wide. This has the same effect as putting the legs apart and can be used in the same way. The lock is terminated by closing the mouth.

4   Either the therapist or client can take and hold information in circuit. Providing both parties are in physical contact, the information is on-line even when held in the therapist's circuit.

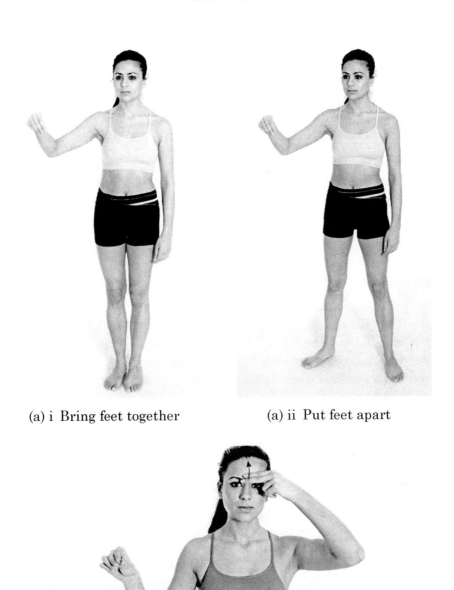

(a) i Bring feet together   (a) ii Put feet apart

(b)   Zip up the glabella

Figure 13.1 Two methods of taking information into circuit lock

It's useful to have both circuit lock methods available. Stroking up the brow is very convenient, but if you are using both of your hands it may be easier to put the feet apart to store the information.

Transferring stored information and *stacking*

It's also possible to transfer the method of storing information from one to the other. If you have put your legs apart to store the information and now need to move your position, you can stroke the brow, allowing you then to bring your legs together and still keep the information in circuit. (There would be no reason I can think of to transfer the information the other way around.)

Combining the two methods makes it possible to store a number of items of information at once. This is called *stacking*. To stack information:

1☐   Take the information into the circuit by putting the legs apart.
2☐   Stroke the brow firmly.
3☐   Bring the legs together.
4☐   Take another piece of information into circuit by putting the legs apart
5☐   Stroke the brow.
6☐   Bring the legs together.
7☐   And so on.

You can stack up to seven pieces of information in this way.

When a number of related issues are *stacked* into the circuit, the corrections chosen by the body can address all of the information that is stacked.

Exercise 13.1 gives you the opportunity to address a specific issue using circuit lock. As always, it's important to *do* the exercise rather than just read it.

Exercise 13.1 Addressing an issue using circuit lock

1   Consider an issue you'd like to work with.
2   Do the pre-checks.
3   Check with the pendulum that you have permission to work with this issue.

4   Think of the issue or say it out loud. As the pendulum gives you a signal change to register the issue, bring your feet together (and your knees if you are sitting down) and then place them at least 18 inches apart. Your issue is now held in the circuit lock.

5   *Optional:* ask your body to confirm that the issue is in circuit lock with an indicator change.

6   With your legs apart, stroke upwards reasonably firmly from the glabella to your hairline. You can now put your feet together and move around.

7   Make a SUD reading for the issue.

8   *Optional:* find the involved emotion (# 12, page 126).

9   Find the priority under-energized meridian by using the alarm points (heavy pressure).

10   Find the priority correction. Do this by using the priority mode and, at the same time, saying the following (the one that produces an indicator change is the priority correction):

   o   Neuro-lymphatic correction
   o   Neuro-vascular correction
   o   Tracing the meridian
   o   Emotional Stress Release (ESR)
   o   Emotional Distress Release (EDR)
   o   Balancing acupoints

11   Do the correction.

12   Firmly touch the under-energized meridian alarm point again. If it still indicates, find the next priority correction (point 10 above).

13   Continue until the alarm point is clear (i.e. heavy pressure on the alarm point does not produce a signal change).

14   Ask if another meridian is needed. If so, proceed from point 9 above.

15   When no further meridians are indicated, tap your brow to cancel the circuit lock.

16   Say your issue again. If you still get a signal change there is more work to be done with this issue. Use the other corrections if you would like to.

17   Notice how you feel about the original issue now, and give it a SUD score. In all probability it will have reduced and may be at zero.   A§

Well done. The mini-balance is very helpful in itself, and it forms the basis of the full self-kinesiology balance.

Summary of the full self-kinesiology balance

The protocol for the full self-kinesiology balance appears quite involved, but what you are doing is actually quite simple. In brief, this is what you are aiming to do:

1☐ Formulate the goal.
2☐ Elicit all the information you need.
3☐ Revisit all the antecedents (contributory factors or sources) of the problem.
4☐ Resolve these experiences.
5☐ With this resolution and your new perception, anticipate and pre-view your future behaviour.

First, the protocol, with each step explained and elucidated. For convenience, the steps are provided, without the notes, in appendix 2.

Notes on the self-kinesiology balance

All of the concepts and procedures of the full balance are already familiar to you. It isn't vital to follow every single step of the protocol on each occasion or do everything exactly as instructed. While you are getting the hang of it you may want to skip the steps designated as *optional*. Whatever you do will be of real benefit.

As you become more familiar with the materials you can gradually expand the balance until you are using the full protocol. Once you become familiar with the whole procedure *and the reasons for each step*, feel free to modify it to suit you. However, I advise working towards using the whole protocol and becoming familiar with it before you experiment with it too much. That way, you ensure you understand it properly first. There are good reasons for each step.

Have an initial read through these notes and then use your pendulum and follow the procedure, working with an issue, to give yourself a self-kinesiology balance.

1   Do the pre-checks and ask permission to address your issue.

The pre-checks should be very familiar to you by now: switching; hydration; zip-up; ionization; hyperstress.

If you don't do the pre-checks you can't be confident that the pendulum's responses are accurate. If you need reminding, see chapter 2 for a full account and appendix 1 (or the beginning of chapter 4) for a summary.

2   Use the pendulum to find and confirm the best wording for your goal.

Make sure that you are working with the priority goal. Then make sure you have exactly the right wording for your goal. Remember that the time taken to formulate the precise wording of your goal is very well spent. By addressing the exact wording you are also formulating the exact nature of the problem and taking your first important step to resolve it (see chapter 12).

3   *Optional:* Find the percentage of stress involved and the available energy to address the issue.

Use the pendulum to take a reading of the percentage stress (zero is no stress; 100 is the most stress imaginable) and available energy (zero is no energy at all to resolve the issue and 100 is all the energy you need) before the balance. This enables you to monitor your progress precisely as you will take another reading at the end of the balance.

4   *Optional:* Identify and acknowledge the primary emotion(s).

Acknowledging the primary emotions can lead to more information about the issue; it also puts the emotion on-line, giving a more complete account of the problem. Use the pendulum and the five-element emotion chart (figure 7.1, page 124) to identify the primary emotions.

5   Ask: *Do I need more information?* If you do, find out what.

By making conscious what's going on and what it means you are able to define the issues clearly, and this helps resolution. All problems are *badly formed*, we learn from NLP; that is to say, they just don't stand up to scrutiny. Often just through clarifying and delimiting the problem it begins to unravel. At all stages of the process ask, *Do I need more information?* The rigorous gathering of information and acknowledgement of the issues will normally take you at least halfway to resolution.

6   Ask: *Am I ready to correct?* If not, find out if you need more information or check that you have permission. Trust whatever comes up.

After your body tells you that you have all the information you need about the issue, ask if you're ready to make the corrections. If not, find out what you need to do first.

7   Ask: *Are there any corrections to be done in present time?* If so, ask: *Do I need a meridian?* If you need a meridian, use the alarm points to find the priority meridian to correct and the correction(s) required. Perform the correction(s) for the meridian.

The correction for a meridian will probably be neuro-lymphatic stimulation, neuro-vascular stimulation or tracing the meridian, but could be anything else. Once you have studied chapter 17 on food and nutrition it may be a food or supplement that you most need to balance the meridian.

To find out which correction will balance the meridian, state the suggested correction (the relevant correction will produce an indicator change); or use the digital finger modes described later in this chapter (the associated mode will produce an indicator change).

8   Ask: *Are there any more corrections in the present?* If so, identify and perform the correction(s).

You should keep asking this question until you have performed all the corrections required in the present.

9   Ask: *Do I have permission to go back in time?* If the answer is no, do F/O holding while thinking through the issue. You can also ask what else you need to do first.

If you do not have permission to go back in time either you are not ready to do so, or doing so is unnecessary. However, most problems are triggered in the present but come from the past, and it is usually necessary to go back in time to resolve the problem completely.

If you don't have permission because your body insists you aren't ready, you may need to do any of the following: (1) find out more information; (2) do more corrections in the present; (3) do F/O holding; or (4) come back to the issue at a later time (because you've done enough for now).

Your intention is to go back to the most appropriate antecedent event that relates to the issue. This may not be the initial cause; and there may be a number of incidents or periods of time to visit and address before the issue is resolved.[5]

10   Once you have permission, go back to the antecedent age. When you reach this age, establish what was happening. If this proves very difficult, ask whether it is necessary to know consciously what was happening. If it is, keep eliciting information until the pendulum agrees that you have all the information you need.

---

5   You know that an issue is resolved when you can't get the problem back, even when you try.

Let the pendulum take you back to the relevant year. You should already know how to do this. Count back in chunks of five or ten years until you get a signal change. Then go through that chunk of years, year by year, until you get a signal change, letting you know the relevant year. When you get to the year, find out what was going on then. Usually you will immediately have an idea about what was going on at this time. Confirm with the pendulum that you have the relevant incident or relationship. If you have difficulties, narrow down the possibilities with guesses, checking with the pendulum until you have all the information you need. It is likely that the relevant experience will flash into your mind. Trust your intuition, even if it doesn't immediately seem relevant or to make sense.

11 *Optional:* Identify the primary emotion(s) and the percentage stress and available energy at this specific age.

This is particularly helpful if you haven't been able to identify the relevant experience. Identifying the primary emotions may help you to identify what was going on at that time.

12 Ask: *Am I ready to correct this?* If not, find out whether you need more information, or if something else is required. When you're ready to correct, ask if you need a meridian, and find it using the alarm points. Correct the meridians in priority order. Then find out what other corrections are required and perform them.

If your body says you're not ready to correct this, find out if you need more information, or try doing ESR or F/O holding to alleviate the associated stress.

After each correction ask if there's more to do, and ask whether you need any more information. Keep doing this until all the required corrections have been done for this age.

13 *Optional:* **Check that the emotion from point 11 above is now clear by restating the emotion. If it is now clear, there will be no signal change. Also re-check the percentage of stressors and available energy pertinent to this age.**

These checks help you to keep you informed of your progress and should encourage you, even if the issue itself does not yet seem different.

14 *Optional:* **Ask:** *Are there other ages to visit?* **If so, ask:** *Backward in time?* **If yes, go backwards in time. If no, ask:** *Forward in time?* **If yes, go forward in time. When you get to the next antecedent age, gather all the information required. Then proceed from point 11 above.**

You are looking for another antecedent incident or period to go back to and resolve, if there is one. *When all antecedent events are resolved, there should be nothing left of the problem.*

15 **Ask permission to return to the present, and ask the pendulum to give you a signal change when you're fully back in the present.**

16 *Optional:* **Recheck the original primary emotion. It should now be clear. Also recheck percentage of stressors (which should have changed and may be at zero) and available energy (which should have changed and may be at 100).**

There is likely to be no signal change when you now restate the primary emotion from point 4 above. This means that the emotion has lost its charge with respect to your issue. If the stressors are not now at zero and the available energy isn't now at 100 per cent, then you may have more work to do on this issue on another occasion. Or it may be that your body will do the remaining processing in its own time, so that if you check the issue again in a week you will find it clear.

17   Ask: *Do I have permission to visit the goal?* If granted, imagine you have now achieved your goal. Using the present tense, describe what it means to you to have achieved it. When you are ready, check with the pendulum that your visit to the goal is complete. Ask permission to return to the present, and for a signal change when you're there.

When you describe what it means to have achieved your goal, you may be describing a perception that's now different, or what is different in your life. As if it has already happened, consider what achieving this goal does for you. This prepares your body to give you what you want. It also gives your body an opportunity to check if there are any other issues that need addressing, and that the goal is as you intended. When you're ready, ask permission and return to the present. Ask the pendulum to give you a signal change when you are back in the present.

18   In the present, restate your goal. If there's a signal change you know there's more work to do.

Lack of signal change implies there is no longer stress attached to achieving your goal. Notice how you now feel in relation to your goal.

19   Ask: *Is there is more work to be done on this issue?* If so, find out when you can come back to it.

You may need to leave some time for your body to process the changes that have been made. You can ask if you need to leave at least one day, two days, and so on; or at least one week, and so on.

20 Finally, thank your body for the work it has done and the changes it has made. Undertake to be responsible for making it happen.

Your body appreciates your thanks. It's simply a matter of respecting yourself. It may be easier to respect yourself when you are addressing that *other* part of yourself, your unconscious. You can't reasonably expect others to thank you, like you or treat you properly, unless you are doing all these to and for yourself. Indeed, nearly always the way others treat us is a reflection of our own attitude to ourselves.

Well done! You have worked through an issue using your own inner therapist communicated through the pendulum.

Troubleshooting

The main problem you are likely to encounter is the pendulum giving you nonsensical results. If this happens, either: (1) you do not have permission to address this issue; or (2) the issue has stressed your body so much that the energy circuits have blown (exercise 13.2).

Always bear in mind that you're working *with* your body. If at any time you feel you're fighting yourself, take a break or do some ESR or F/O holding. Remember that your body will always be trying to help you, even if this doesn't seem like the case. Work with whatever comes up – even if it seems like a detour. If blocks emerge, address them (don't fight them).

Exercise 13.2 Troubleshooting

1 Check the central meridian energy by zipping up (no signal change) and zipping down (signal change). If you get reversed results, do the correction (meridian flush or harmonizing posture).
2 Check for switching: touch the K27s (either side of the sternum below the clavicle); touch the ends of the central and governing meridians (under the nose and just below your bottom lip); and touch the coccyx. If any of these produce a signal change, do the correction (rub the points while placing a hand over the navel).
3 Check for hydration. Say *Water*. If you get a signal change, drink some pure water.
4 Ask whether you have permission to address this issue.

5   Finally, perhaps you don't understand what your body is trying to say;
         ask the pendulum to find another way of communicating the body's
         wishes.

Digital finger modes

Finger modes provide a useful way of organizing and applying corrections
(figure 13.2). We have already come across one or two finger modes. They are
a non-verbal method of communicating directly with the body. It is not quite
clear how they work. Perhaps they are simply a way of clarifying intention;
but it is claimed that they are more than this: that fingers have energy flows
corresponding to different functions. Bruce Dewe MD, a leading proponent
and developer of kinesiology and creator of the Professional Kinesiology
Practitioner (PKP) programme, reports that different people independently
came up with the same finger modes to represent a specific correction.[6]

Applied Kinesiology (the system pioneered by George Goodheart) maintains
that finger modes are more reliable than verbal questioning. Whether this
is true or not, finger modes provide a useful adjunct to help communications
with the body. The four basic finger modes (figure 13.2) were discovered by
Alan Beardall in 1983.

You can use the finger modes, or you can use the verbal category headings; it
doesn't matter (table 13.1). When you are ready to make a correction, apply
the four digital finger modes, one at a time (or verbally state the categories);
a signal change means that a correction in that category will be useful. Find
the specific correction.

You can also use the priority mode (middle finger tip to thumb crease); but
using both finger modes while holding the pendulum is tricky! To solve this,
either (1) hold the priority mode while stating the categories verbally; (2)
have an *intention* of finding the priority while holding the digital finger
modes; or (3) put priority mode into circuit with circuit lock (figure 13.1).

You will notice that there is very little under the category of *biochemical* in
table 13.1 (page 224). We have addressed the importance of hydration but we

---

6   PKP uses finger modes extensively, each finger having at least 20 different
possible modes.

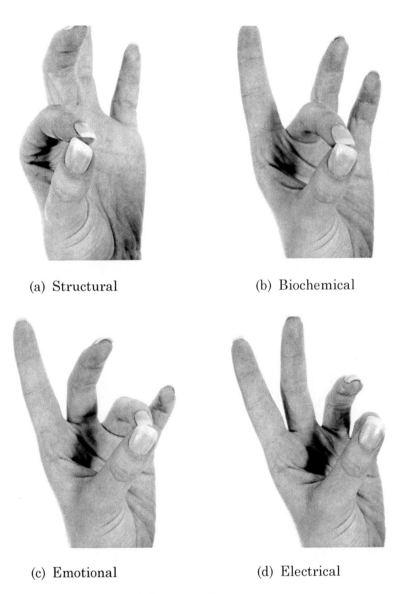

(a) Structural   (b) Biochemical

(c) Emotional   (d) Electrical

Figure 13.2 Digital finger modes

have not yet considered nutrition. Nutrition is an important part of kinesiology; it is one of the four dimensions. We shall address it in part III.

We have not yet made any directly structural corrections, and this column in the table is empty. In fact, kinesiology is very concerned with posture and muscle balance. This dimension is not fully realized in this text simply

Electrical

#	Electrical	TEST	CORRECTION
1	Auditory perception	66	66
2	Visual perception	68	69
3	Brain integration (cross-crawl)	78	78
4	Brain integration (cross-crawl) with eye movements	–	81
5	Tracing the lemmiscate (vision)	–	82
6	Tracing the lemmiscate (writing)	–	84
7	Gait reflexes	84	85
16	Tracing the meridian	–	163
17	Acupoints to tonify and sedate	–	164
18	Central & governing hook-up	–	171
19	Time of day balance	–	173
20	Balancing acupoints	–	174
21	Tracing a meridian backwards (for pain)	–	177

Emotional

#	Emotional	TEST	CORRECTION
8	Emotional stress release (ESR)	91	91
9	Frontal/Occipital holding	–	98
10	Emotional Distress Release (EDR)	–	99
11	Colour balance	–	101
12	Acknowledging the involved emotion	–	126
15	Neuro-vascular (NV) reflexes	161	161

Biochemical

#	Biochemical	TEST	CORRECTION
14	Neuro-lymphatic (NL) reflexes	154	157

Structural

#	Structural	TEST	CORRECTION

Other methods

#		TEST	CORRECTION
13	Identifying the antecedents of an issue	–	131
22	Working with life choices	–	186
23	Modelling a third-person perspective	–	186
24	Generating a support system	–	189
25	Giving the problem back (1)	–	197

Notes:

(i) When the unconscious body tells you that you're ready to make a correction, form the digital finger modes one at a time. An indicator change means that a correction from this category is required. Go down the list, using the correction numbers or stating the name of the correction to find the required correction.

(ii) The Biochemical category will have to wait for chapter 17. The Structural category has no corrections yet, but will be needed in the next chapter.

Table 13.1 Tests & corrections according to finger-mode category (& other correction methods)

because our tool is the pendulum rather than the muscle test. Nevertheless, the techniques here not only balance the meridians but help improve posture. For more explicit help with posture and structural aspects, I recommend a visit to a kinesiologist (check that they do postural muscle balancing) or learn Touch for Health.

Part III

THE PATH
TO FULL HEALTH

Part III

14

Healing Body & Soul

In this chapter a number of highly effective kinesiology techniques[1] are described. Their order isn't important. Any of them may be helpful for any problem, even if sometimes you can't see their relevance. Try them out. Once your unconscious body has experienced a correction, it can be added to your repertoire when you give yourself a balance or address a problem.

Of course it may be that your body does not need the particular correction. The great thing about kinesiology is that it can only do you good – it can't do you any harm. So perform the correction to become familiar with it, even if your body doesn't need it. Performing the correction helps your body to understand what the correction does, enabling it to choose this correction when it's needed in the future.

Tip:

> You can ask your body to recall a time when you needed the correction. *Say:* Go back to a time when I needed this correction and give me an indicator change when I'm there. Your body will give you an indicator change, showing that it has re-established a state when the correction was required. *Doing this will incidentally help you to heal something from the past (even though you won't consciously know what it is).*

---

1   With the exception of # 34, all of the corrections in this chapter come from Three In One Concepts, developed by Gordon Stokes and Daniel Whiteside. I have retained the Three In One Concepts names of the corrections – although I understand that these are currently under review. See the qualifying remarks about the inclusion of these corrections in the preface (page xxiv).

Each technique includes the following:

- ○ The name of the correction.
- ○ The general finger mode category to which it belongs (electrical, emotional, biochemical, structural).
- ○ A specific finger mode (where given).
- ○ Information about the correction.
- ○ The test.
- ○ The correction.

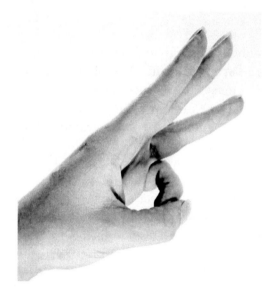

Figure 14.1 Body polarity finger mode

Body polarity

Category: **electrical**
Specific finger mode: **thumb over little fingernail (see figure 14.1)**

This very important correction helps to ensure the electrical polarity of your body is harmonized. Every part of the body has an electrical charge. Muscles have a charge in the same way as cells do. Different sides of the body have a different charge. The front of the body on the right side has a positive charge; the front left side has a negative charge. The back of the body on the right side has a negative charge; the back left side has a positive charge. On the right hand the palm has a positive charge; the forefinger is positive; the middle finger is negative; the ring finger is positive; the little finger is negative. On the left hand the palm is negative; the forefinger is negative; the middle finger is positive; and so on (see figure 14.2). This is why we use two adjoining fingers to produce a neutral touch. The thumbs are neutral.

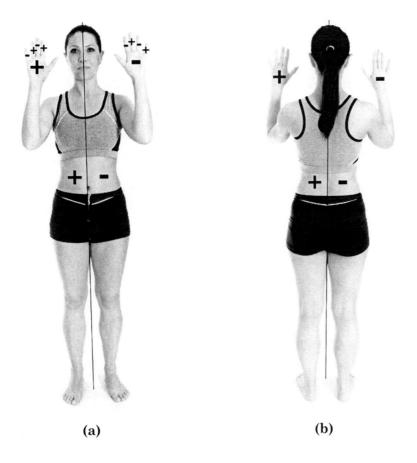

(a)   (b)

Figure 14.2 Body polarity map

When a muscle is contracted, the belly of the muscle has a negative charge and the ends of the muscle (the origin and insertion) have a positive charge. When you place your left forefinger (negatively charged) on the belly of a contracted muscle, you are putting negative to negative: the two are repelled, giving a signal change showing stress (or an unlocking muscle in muscle testing). If you place your left middle finger (positively charged) in the belly of a contracted muscle, the two will attract each other, and there will be no indicator change (the muscle would remain locked in muscle testing). Using a pendulum, most people will get a signal change when you put a positive to a positive or negative to a negative (indicating stress).

When a muscle is in extension, the polarity is the opposite: the belly of the muscle has a positive charge and the ends a negative charge.

Test this, if you like. Do the pre-tests first, of course. With the pendulum in your right hand, lift up your knee. With your left index finger (negative charge) touch the middle of your contracted thigh muscle (your quadriceps, halfway between knee and hip). (If the polarity of your body is in order you are applying negative to negative; this will produce a signal change.) Touch with your left middle finger. (You are applying positive to negative; there will be no signal change.) Put your knee down and test again with the muscle in extension (relaxed). The results should be the opposite.

When this correction is required, it may mean you are out of touch with significant parts of yourself. The correction helps to re-establish wholeness.

26 TEST
Body polarity

You can use either test or both: point 1 is the simplest, but point 2 gives you more information about what the test is about.

1▢   Hold the body polarity finger mode (figure 14.1, page 230). If you get a signal change, perform the correction.
2▢   Place the pads of the fingertips and thumbs together (tip of thumb to tip of thumb; tip of forefinger to tip of forefinger, and so on). Take this into circuit by putting the feet (and knees, if you are sitting down) together and apart. Have the pendulum swing on the YES/POSITIVE axis. If it moves from there directly to the NO/STRESSED axis, the correction is required. If body polarity is correct, since the same fingers of both hands have opposite polarities, the body would be comfortable in this position and there would be no indicator change.[2]

---

2   Religious figures (and smug politicians) often adopt this posture which represents balance.

26 CORRECTION
Body polarity

1☐   Hold your ESR points and take this into circuit by putting your legs
      apart. Keep ESR in circuit as you perform the correction.
2☐   Using two fingers of your right hand deeply massage the K27 point
      (the end of your kidney meridian, at the side of the sternum just below
      the clavicle) on the *right* side of your body for 20–30 seconds.
3☐   *At the same time*, using two fingers of your left hand deeply massage
      the K27 on the *left* side.
4☐   Repeat the initial test. It should now be clear (no signal change).

Unthinking responses: Common Integrative Area (CIA)

Category: structural

When affected by stress the body will revert to automatic responses used
habitually in the past. The value of this is that you don't have to think about
your response, your body just does it. The disadvantage is that the automatic
response is probably outmoded and inappropriate.

27 TEST
Common Integrative Area (CIA)

1☐   Holding the pendulum with one hand, with the other use four fingers
      to tap behind the *left* ear, above the mastoid process (level with the top
      of the ear) a few times and then touch and hold that point and observe
      whether you get a signal change.
2☐   If you get no signal change, repeat on the other side of the head, behind
      the *right* ear.
3☐   If you get a signal change on either side, stress is leading you to react
      to current challenges with habitual modes of behaviour rather than
      responding creatively in the present. Perform the correction.

When in stress, the body stands to attention and becomes rigid, restricting
and confining energy flow. Soldiers on parade have been known to collapse

from standing rigidly in one position. The correction provides a means of freeing the muscles which have tensed up and become rigid, locking the whole system. As the system unlocks you are once again back in a place of choice and, instead of rigid thought, flexibility is returned.

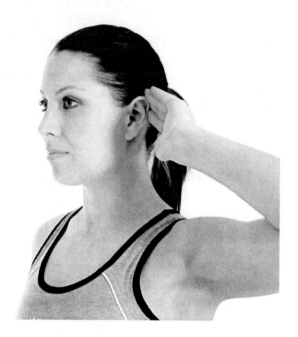

Figure 14.3   CIA test

27 CORRECTION
Common Integrative Area (CIA)

1☐   Firmly pluck the Achilles tendon above each heel a number of times.
2☐   Firmly pluck the hamstring tendons on the back of each knee a number of times, and just above the back of the knee.
3☐   Stand up and let your left arm hang down freely. With the right hand firmly grasp the top of the shoulder (the upper trapezius muscle) on your left – the fleshy part between the neck and shoulder joint. Hold the muscle firmly to prevent it moving while you rotate the shoulder joint in small circles forwards and backwards. Swap arms and repeat.
4☐   Repeat the initial test: tap behind the ear and maintain the touch. The test should now be clear (no signal change).

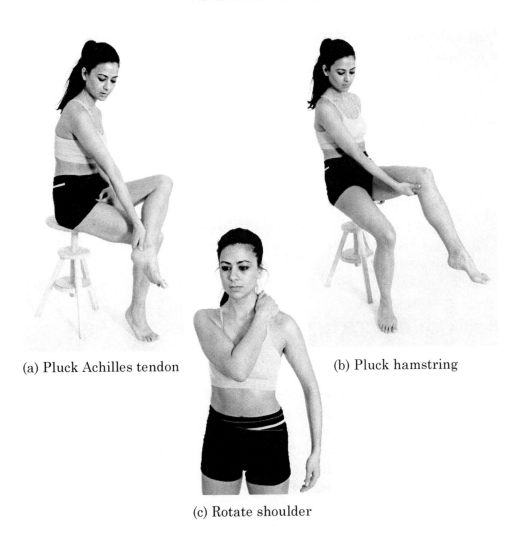

(a) Pluck Achilles tendon   (b) Pluck hamstring

(c) Rotate shoulder

Figure 14.4   CIA correction

Out of the darkness: fixation

Category: structural

Darkness is associated with fear, pain and sadness; loss of connection with the living world of the day and an emersion into the lifeless, subterranean world of the night. This correction brings light to the brain, specifically the pituitary gland, helping the eyes to renew their motion and come out of their state of fixation, immobility and darkness. This correction can also help you if you suffer from SAD (Seasonal Affective Disorder).

28 TEST
Fixation

1☐ Hold a sheet of black paper or card (or anything coloured black) about ten or twelve inches or so (25 or 30 cm) from your eyes.

2☐ If you get a signal change, perform the correction. (*Note:* hold the pendulum up high so that you can see any signal change while looking at the black paper.)

28 CORRECTION
Fixation

1☐ Shine a torchlight on the glabella (the point between the eyebrows, just above the bridge of the nose) until you get an indicator change confirming the correction is complete. This will be between five seconds and one minute, depending on the need and the brightness of the torch.

2☐ Ask the pendulum if you need to visit the past. If you do, go back to the age indicated and repeat the correction at that age. Continue visiting the past as long as the pendulum indicates there are past ages to go back to.

3☐ Return to the present (say: *Take me back to the present and give me an indicator change to confirm when I am there*). When you're in the present, again look at the sheet of black paper. There should now be no indicator change.

Adrenal stress

Category: **biochemical**

This test reveals whether you have no adrenal stress or adrenal stress that is *minor*, *significant* or *major*. The correction for all three levels is the same.

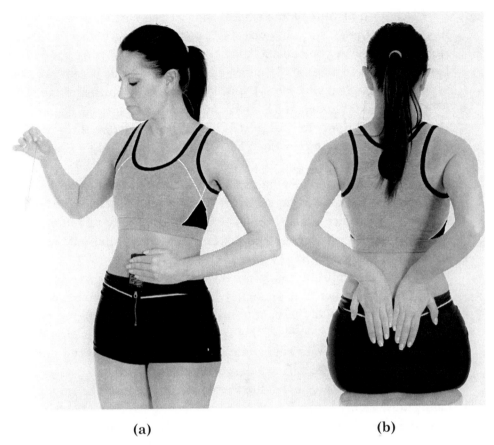

(a)   (b)

Figure 14.5 Test for *minor* adrenal stress

29 TEST
Adrenal stress

1⊓   With the pendulum swinging on the YES–POSITIVE axis, hold some
     refined sugar near the navel (or imagine eating refined sugar) (figure
     14.5 a). This should be stressful to the body and you should get a change
     of swing to NO–STRESSED axis. If pendulum swings to NO, go to point
     2 below. If there is no change of swing and it remains on the YES axis,
     go to point 3 below.

2⊓   If the pendulum has changed its swing to NO–STRESSED axis, this
     means the sugar (or thought of the sugar) has stressed your body – as
     it ought to. Find out whether you have *minor* adrenal stress or not.

Place both of your palms side by side at the bottom of your back, fingers pointing down (see figure 14.5, page 237). With your hands in this position (over your adrenals) take it into circuit by bringing your feet together and at least 18 inches apart. Pick up your pendulum and start it swinging on your YES–POSITIVE axis. If it changes to the NO–STRESSED axis this means there is *minor* adrenal stress. The rest of the test doesn't apply to you: *go straight to the correction.* If the pendulum remains swinging on the YES–POSITIVE axis, that's great: you are adrenal-stress free and no correction is necessary.

3☐ If there is no change of swing in point 1 above the implication is that your body wants refined sugar to give it some energy. *It shouldn't want refined sugar.* Since it does, this means that your body has *significant* stress; it wants a boost of energy from the sugar. Find out whether your stress is *significant* or *major*.

With your pendulum swinging on the YES–POSITIVE axis, imagine eating some fruit (such as an apple). Your body should have a positive response to fruit and the pendulum should remain swinging on the same YES–POSITIVE axis. If this is the case, the stress is *significant* but not major. It wants sugar but is also happy to have the natural sugars provided by fruit. Go to the correction.

If the idea of eating fruit stressed the body and the pendulum changed its swing to the NO–STRESSED axis, go to point 4 below.

4☐ The idea of eating fruit is stressful to the body. It wants refined sugar now – it doesn't want to bother with digesting fruit! This means that your body is in *major* stress. Go to the correction.

The correction is the same whatever the degree of stress.

29 CORRECTION
Adrenal stress

1☐ With two fingers very gently hold the posterior fontanel – a point just in front of the crown of your head.

2☐ While holding the point on your head, with two fingers and the thumb of your other hand massage one inch above and either side of your navel.

3☐ Swap hands and repeat. (See figure 14.6.)

4☐   This correction brings extra energy to your adrenals. Re-test.

5☐   Most important: find out where the stress is coming from (chapter 11 will help) and address this – especially if you are suffering from major stress.

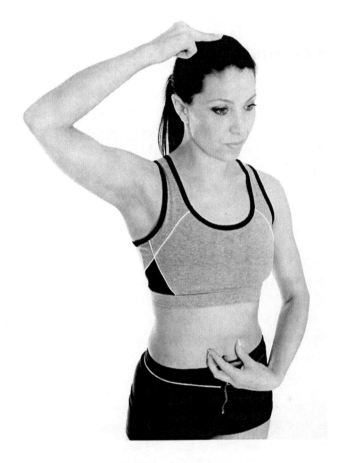

Figure 14.6 Adrenal stress correction

Breathing: constricted cranials

Category: **structural**

The cranial plates of the skull are designed to move as we breathe but, as a result of stress and restricted breathing, these plates can become locked.

When they become locked the brain is not able to function fully, preventing the forebrain (the part of the brain responsible for human intelligence) from working properly.[3]

30 TEST
Constricted cranials

1☐ Neutral touch governing meridian (vessel) 20 (GV 20). This point is on the top of the head. If you imagine a vertical line from the orifice of each ear to the top of your head, GV 20 is just behind where the line reaches the top of the head (figure 14.7).

2☐ If you get an indicator change when you touch GV 20, do the correction.

30 CORRECTION
Constricted cranials

The correction is to hold GV 20 while rubbing neuro-lymphatic (NL) points and holding neuro-vascular (NV) points. If you had five hands you would simply hold GV 20 while at the same time you would (1) hold the jaw points,

---

3 Efficient breathing occurs in the abdomen, not the chest. However, breathing should be slight; many health problems, including asthma, can be caused by inefficient over-breathing ('hyperventilation'):

> Hyperventilation causes a depletion of carbon dioxide; low levels of carbon dioxide in the organism cause blood vessels to spasm and also cause oxygen starvation of the tissues. This results in a whole range of 'defence mechanisms' that have been previously misunderstood and labelled as diseases. It was not difficult to surmise that vessel spasming occurring in hypertension could occur also with other types of diseases, for example: stenocardia (angina pectoris) with the resultant myocardial infarction (heart attack): end arteritis (inflammation of the innermost coat of an artery, usually occurring in legs) or ulcerative stomach disease. (Buteyko Health Centre. Taken from www.buteyko.com.)

The health dangers of deep breathing are elucidated by Dr Konstantin Buteyko, and would seem to be contrary to received wisdom. Buteyko breathing methods have also found to be helpful for people suffering from allergies, bronchitis and general breathing problems. One client reported that it helped her ME.

and (2) massage the collarbone points. Since you only have two hands (hope-fully), you will take points into your body's circuit.

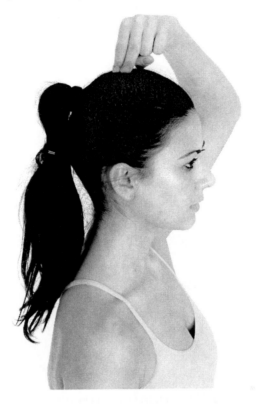

Figure 14.7 Location of GV 20

1⌐ Locate the points on the jaw. They are on the cheeks, where you can feel that the upper and lower gums meet (figure 14.8, page 242). Hold these two points for a few seconds and put them into your body's circuit by bringing your feet (and knees if you are sitting down) together and apart. Keep them in circuit.

2⌐ With two fingers of one hand, hold GV 20 very gently.

3⌐ Keep holding GV 20 while you massage the NL points under the middle of each clavicle (see figure 14.8) for 20 seconds or so while touching GV 20. Massage one side first, and then the other.

4⌐ Bring your feet together to close the circuit and re-test by holding GV 20. If it is clear, your job is done; if it still indicates, continue with the corrections below.

5⌐ Gently touch GV 20 and put your feet (and knees) together and apart, taking the point into circuit. Keep this in circuit.

6☐ With two fingers of each hand hold the jaw points gently for 30 seconds or so or (preferably) until the pulses synchronize. Close the circuit.

7☐ Use the pendulum and touch GV 20 again. This time it should be clear (no signal change).

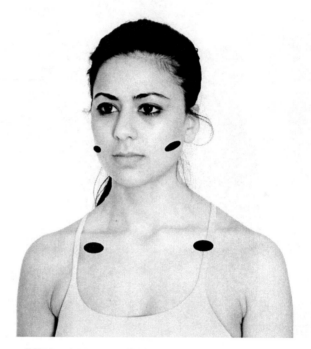

Figure 14.8 Constricted cranials correction points

Oneness: cloacal energy

Category: **electrical**

The *cloaca* relates to an early part of foetal development, just a few weeks after conception. At this time there is no real differentiation between the upper part of the body, constituting the early formation of the brain, eyes and ears, and the lower part of the body, constituting the elementary processes of digestion, reproduction and elimination.

During this time no real distinction exists between the processes and functions of the body. The sacrum and the cranium are integrated and connected. This is a time of wholeness and oneness, with no separation of thinking and feeling, mind and body, spirit and sexuality. Although this stage of development is only very brief (a matter of weeks), the body registers everything.

When confronted with stress, reproductive functions cease to work well, affecting sexual function and desire and menstruation; and the digestive system is thrown out of rhythm. There may be a feeling of separation from oneness and of alienation from the body itself. The result of all this is depletion of energy.

The cranium and sacrum are connected by a number of circuits. The connection points are as follows.

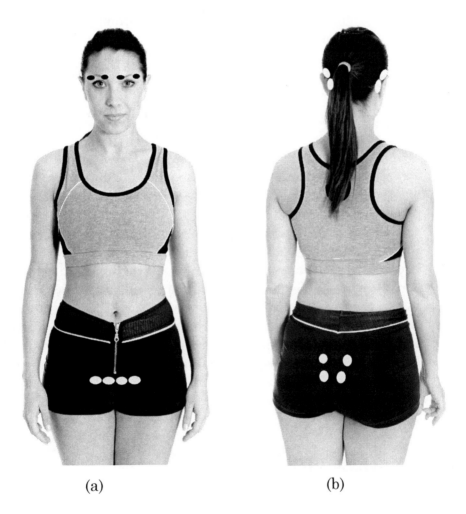

(a)   (b)

Figure 14.9 The cloacal points

     ○   On the upper front of the body on the bony ridge of the socket above the eye

     ○   On the upper back of the body: immediately behind the ear. The area extends from level with the top of the ear above the mastoid process to level with the bottom of the ear on the mastoid process.

     ○   On the lower front of the body: on the pubic bone.

     ○   On the lower back of the body: near the bottom of the sacrum, just either side of the midline.

The correction involves reconnecting the upper and lower body. Points on the upper body connect to points on the lower body, front and back, left and right, in any combination. You will find the priority circuits that need to be reconnected.

31 TEST
Cloacal energy

1☐   Say *Cloacals*; or touch the bony ridge of the socket above the eye. If you get an indicator change, find the disconnected energy circuits (as detailed below).

2☐   Put priority mode in circuit; or simply have the *intention* of finding the priority circuits as you carry out the following test.

3☐   Touch (with two fingers) along the ridges of the socket above each eye and the points behind each ear until you get an indicator change. This is your priority upper point (figure 14.9, page 243).

4☐   As the pendulum registers an indicator change, put your legs together and apart to take this point into circuit.

5☐   Find the priority lower point by touching (with two fingers) the points along the pubic bone and on the sacrum (figure 14.9). The priority point will produce an indicator change.

31 CORRECTION
Cloacal energy

1☐   Hold the priority upper and lower points with minimum pressure for at least 30 seconds or until the pulses synchronize.

2☐   Find any further sets of points in the same way: touch the upper points until you get a signal change and take into circuit; touch the lower points until you get a signal change. Hold the points until the pulses synchronize.

3☐   Continue (if necessary) until all the points are done and when you say *cloacals* there is no signal change.

Note that the points behind the ears relate to hearing; the points above the eyes relate to seeing; the points on the pubic bone relate to sexuality; and the points on the sacrum relate to past denials of goals. If you are able to identify the issues involved with each point the correction will be even more effective.

Energy: RNA/DNA

Category: **biochemical**

This correction helps to re-energize the body and may improve memory and counter dyslexia.

32 TEST
RNA/DNA

1☐   Touch the glabella (between the eyebrows at the top of the nose) with two fingers.

2☐   If you get a signal change, perform the correction.

Read carefully through the correction before you perform it. It involves putting yourself into a light trance – which is perfectly easy to do. There is nothing special about the wording in point 5 of the correction. Get the general idea and make it up yourself. Spend a few minutes reading and preparing what you will say to yourself. It won't be helpful to your trance if you're reading at the time!

32 CORRECTION
RNA/DNA

1☐   Sit or lie down. If seated, it's preferable if you can lean your head back. If lying down, lie on your back and put a cushion under the backs of your knees.

2☐   *(Optional)* Apply F/O holding while you complete the correction; or put F/O holding in circuit.

3☐   *(Optional)* Apply trance finger mode:[4] tip of middle finger to halfway between the tip of the thumb and the inside of the middle crease (figure 14.10). You can hold this mode throughout the correction or put it into circuit.[5]

4☐   Put yourself into a light trance by bringing your focus in to your body. After closing your eyes, first notice what's going on *outside* of you: specifically any sounds. Notice how your body feels *on the surface*: the temperature on your skin; the pressure of your clothes; the weight of your body. Pay attention to your *muscles*. How relaxed are you? Which muscles are more relaxed than others? Allow your body to relax. Pay attention to your *breathing*. Notice how it becomes more rhythmic as you relax. Attend to how you are feeling *emotionally*. Notice any feelings in your chest or abdomen that accompany your emotions.

5☐   Let go of all of this and imagine a warm, healing, golden light shining through the crown of your head and into your body . . . Feel the warmth of this healing light internally, as it shines into every part of your body, especially any dark areas, healing and restoring you. Flowing into your lungs and heart . . . As the light penetrates your body, sense the energy that it brings, as all of the organs of your body are bathed in this healing, revitalizing glow . . . Feel the light flowing into your organs of digestion and reproduction . . . And down into your legs and feet and toes . . . And along your arms, into your hands and fingers . . . Feel it in your head, your brain, and your face . . . Feel it in all your muscles, revitalizing, nourishing and healing . . . As the energizing

---

4   This finger mode, along with the pendulum mode (figure 2.4) and totality mode (figure 18.1), my unconscious revealed to me during a walk with my wife in Queen's Park (the park itself) in north-west London in 2001.

5   Do you remember how to stack more than a single piece of information into circuit? You can stroke up the brow from between the eyebrows to the hairline, allowing you to stack another piece of information by putting your legs apart (see chapter 13, page 212).

light flows into every cell of your body, recharging your body, notice how your whole body is renewed and regenerated . . .

6☐ Bring yourself gently back to an awareness of the present and your surroundings.

7☐ Ask your body if you need to repeat this exercise, and if so, how often and when. Find out whether there is a particular time of day when it would be most beneficial; find out when this is.

8☐ Touch the glabella again. This time there should be no signal change.

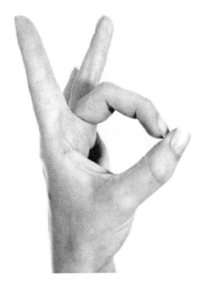

Figure 14.10 Trance finger mode[6]

Emotional rigidity

Category: structural

Specific finger mode: forefinger tightly curled against thumb (figure 14.11)

This simple and effective correction will help if you are prone to be inflexible, or if you deny your feelings and sacrifice yourself. Such inflexibility can give rise to a stiff neck – the physical representation of emotional rigidity.

---

6 My definition of trance is *communicating directly with the unconscious.* So this finger mode helps you to talk directly to your unconscious.

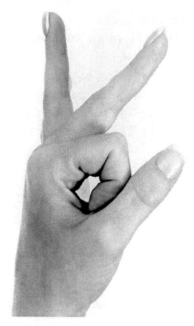

Figure 14.11 Emotional rigidity mode

33 TEST
Emotional rigidity

1☐   Apply the emotional rigidity finger mode.
2☐   If you get a signal change, perform the correction.

33 CORRECTION
Emotional rigidity

The correction involves releasing tension in the neck through isometric exercises. You will be leaning your head and pressing back towards your hand.

1☐   Lean your head to the *left* (so that your ear is closer to your shoulder). Put your right palm against the *right* side of your head. Take a breath and push your head sideways against your hand, while exerting pressure to prevent the head from moving back to an upright position.
2☐   Repeat, leaning your head a little further down to the left.

3⌐   Do this while leaning your head to the right.
4⌐   Repeat, leaning your head a little further down to the right.
5⌐   Lean your head forward and put one hand behind your head. Take a
     breath and push back against your hand.
6⌐   Repeat, leaning your head further forward.
7⌐   Lean your head back and put your palm over your forehead. Take a
     breath and apply pressure to attempt to bring your chin towards your
     chest.
8⌐   Repeat, leaning your head further backwards.

If you habitually deny your feelings, you might want to do something about
it, since acknowledging and appropriately expressing your feelings is the key
to health and happiness.

People who habitually deny their feelings tend to have comparatively smaller
irises (when looked at in relation to the sclera, or white outer coat of the eye).
If this is you, see if the correction enlarges your irises.

Find out what stops you from expressing your emotions and resolve this with
a full balance. You can ask the pendulum:

1⌐   Does this derive from traumas (any unresolved problem experi-
     ence)?
2⌐   Does this problem belong to my parent(s)?

If it derives from traumas, use the pendulum to revisit the traumas and
resolve them, using the techniques in this book. If it is your parents' problem,
acknowledge that this is not your problem and belongs to your parents.

34 CORRECTION
Giving the problem back (2) [7]

1⌐   Identify the problem that belongs to your parent(s) rather than you. It
     might, for example, be fear of expressing anger; inhibition in express-
     ing sexuality; the need to be invisible; not being okay to express emo-
     tion; and so on.

---

7   Also see # 25, Giving the problem back (1), page 197.

2☐   EITHER: Symbolically return the problem to your parent(s) in your imagination. You might think of particular instances where you have exhibited the problem. Give these instances back to your parent(s). It might help to represent the problems with some kind of object, symbol or substance, and return that to your parent(s).
OR: If you would prefer not to give the problem back to your parent(s), throw it away (in your imagination) into the sea; bury it deep under the ground; or send it hurtling into outer space.

3☐   Get some help from a mentor. Your mentor can be imaginary or real; someone you know or don't know personally. Let your unconscious come up with someone now. Let this mentor be a cheerleader for your expression of the desired behaviour. Imagine yourself in a number of different situations where you'd like to express this desired behaviour. Be there, in your imagination, expressing yourself fully, with this support.

4☐   Imagine what life would be like growing up without these inhibitions. Think about how you would be, and imagine you are actually like that, behaving in the way you would like. Imagine it from inside your own body – expressing your feelings freely (and appropriately). This is the real you. This is how you are without your parents' problem.

Remember that *all* emotions are legitimate. It's *behaviour* that needs to be censored and controlled, not emotions. Acknowledging the emotion gives you control over your behaviour – whereas simply trying to censor the behaviour without acknowledging the emotion that gives rise to it is perilous and likely to fail. Reclaim your emotions! Allow yourself to *feel* unreasonably. Choose to *express* those emotions in appropriate ways.

A§ Digestion: ileocaecal valve & Houston valve imbalance

Category: structural

The ileocaecal valve regulates flow from the small intestine (responsible for the assimilation of nutrients from food) to the large intestine. It prevents the contents of the large intestine flowing back into the small intestine. The Houston valve regulates the final section of the large intestine, from the sigmoid colon to the rectum, which affects the need to defecate. Both the ileocaecal valve and the Houston valve should be in balance for the system of the body to be working effectively.

Digestion, as you may be aware, is a precarious business. In our culture constipation is very common; and so are loose bowels, bloating and other problems associated with irritable bowel syndrome (IBS). Eating refined foods (and not enough roughage) is unhelpful. So is stress. The frustrated fight–flight response is particularly upsetting to digestion. If you are continually in a state of fight or flight, your digestion doesn't get a chance to operate properly (the body doesn't want to be bothered with digesting food in the middle of a perceived emergency).

Elimination is sometimes about *letting go*. If constipation is a problem, ask yourself if there's anything you're not letting go of. Small intestine problems can relate to issues with assimilating the things that are nurturing and good for you and differentiating these from what is unwholesome. Again, check out these possibilities using the pendulum. You know how to do it.

Although the large intestine relates to the large intestine meridian, problems with the ileocaecal valve and the Houston valve relate to imbalances in the kidney meridian.

35 TEST
Ileocaecal valve & Houston valve imbalance

1☐　Place both hands (one on top of the other) over the ileocaecal valve, located halfway between your navel and your hip on your right side. With your hands here, put your feet (and knees, if you're sitting) together and apart, to take it into circuit. Keep your legs apart.

2☐　Pick up the pendulum and deliberately start it swinging on the YES/POSITIVE axis. If it immediately switches to the NO/STRESSED axis, the ileocaecal valve requires a correction. Put your feet (and knees) together.

3☐　Put both your hands (one on top of the other) over the Houston valve, located halfway between your navel and your hip on your left side. Put your legs apart to take this into circuit.

4☐　Pick up the pendulum and deliberately swing it on the YES axis. If it immediately switches to the NO/STRESSED axis, the Houston valve requires a correction. Put your feet (and knees) together.

35 CORRECTION
Ileocaecal valve & Houston valve imbalance

1☐   First, put the issue into circuit. To do this, put both hands over the valve that requires a correction and put your feet (and knees if sitting) together and apart. The issue is now in circuit. Keep your legs apart.

2☐   Find out whether the kidney meridian is under- or over-energized. For this, you are going to use the kidney alarm point (at the tip of the floating twelfth rib; see figure 9.3, page 148, for a reminder of its location) *on the same side of the body as the problem* – that is, use the kidney alarm point on the right side of the body for the ileocaecal valve; and use the kidney alarm point on the left side of the body for the Houston valve. (Be careful as you position yourself for this that the movement of your body doesn't accidentally create an indicator change.)

     (i)   With two fingers, very lightly touch the kidney alarm point on the relevant side of the body. If you get a signal change, there is *over-energy*. Go straight to point 3 below.

     (ii)   If there is no signal change, with a neutral touch, using two fingers, touch the same alarm point with heavy pressure. If there is a signal change, there is *under-energy*. Go straight to point 4 below.

3☐   If there is over-energy (signal change on light touch), to correct it you will need to find and correct the *under*-energized meridian.

     (i)   You will already have your legs apart holding the issue (ileocaecal or Houston valve) in circuit. Stroke your brow firmly from glabella to hairline; *or* open your mouth wide until you complete (ii) below. Bring your legs together. You will still have the issue in circuit.

     (ii)   Touch the kidney meridian alarm point again very lightly and, as you get a signal change, put your feet (and knees if you're sitting) together and apart to take the over-energy into circuit. Keep your feet apart. (If you like, you can stroke upwards on your forehead to keep this in circuit, allowing you to put your legs together.)

     (iii)   Now go through the alarm points again (figure 9.3, page 148) to find the under-energized meridian. Touch each alarm point with heavy pressure. If more than one indicates, find the priority.

     (iv)   Stimulate the neuro-lymphatic points (figure 10.1, page 156) for this meridian. Put your feet together.

     (v)   Re-test the under-energized alarm point by touching it again with a heavy touch. If it's clear (no signal change) go to point vii below. If it indicates, take it into circuit by putting your feet apart as the pendulum changes its swing. Stimulate the neuro-vascular points (figure 10.3, page 160) for this meridian. Put your feet together.

(vi) Re-test the under-energized alarm point. If it's clear, go to point vii. If it still indicates, put your feet apart to take into circuit. Trace the meridian (figure 9.1, pages 136–41).

(vii) Put your feet together and tap your brow (if necessary) to close the circuits. Re-test the kidney alarm point (light touch). It should now be clear. Go to point 5 below.

4⌐ If there is under-energy (signal change on heavy touch), take the following steps to correct. *Correct only on the side of the body that indicated a problem* – that is, correct the points on the right side of the body for ileocaecal valve; correct the points on the left side of the body for Houston valve. (See page 154: figure 14.12a for the ileocaecal valve; and 14.12b for the Houston valve.)

(i) You will already have your legs apart holding the issue in circuit. Stroke your brow firmly from glabella to hairline; *or* open your mouth wide until you complete (ii) below. Bring your legs together. You will still have the issue in circuit.

(ii) Touch the kidney alarm point with heavy pressure and, as the signal changes, put your feet (and knees if you're sitting) together and apart. Either keep your legs apart or, to make things easier, stroke upwards on your forehead so that you can put your legs together but still have the under-energized meridian in circuit.

(iii) With a neutral touch hold the following two points at the same time: lung 8 (on the thumb-side of the wrist) and kidney 7 (halfway between the bottom of the calf muscle and the ankle bone). If the problem is on the right side (ileocaecal), hold kidney 7 on your right leg with two fingers of your *right* hand while holding lung 8 (on right hand) with two fingers of your *left* hand. Reverse hands if the problem is the Houston valve. Hold the points for 30 seconds or until the pulses synchronize.

(iv) Massage the front of the shoulder and halfway between navel and hip (20 seconds).

(v) With a light neutral touch, hold the following two points simultaneously: governing vessel (GV) 21 (in the middle of the top of the head) and stomach (St) 25 (an inch to the side of the navel). (Hold for 30 seconds or until the pulses synchronize.)

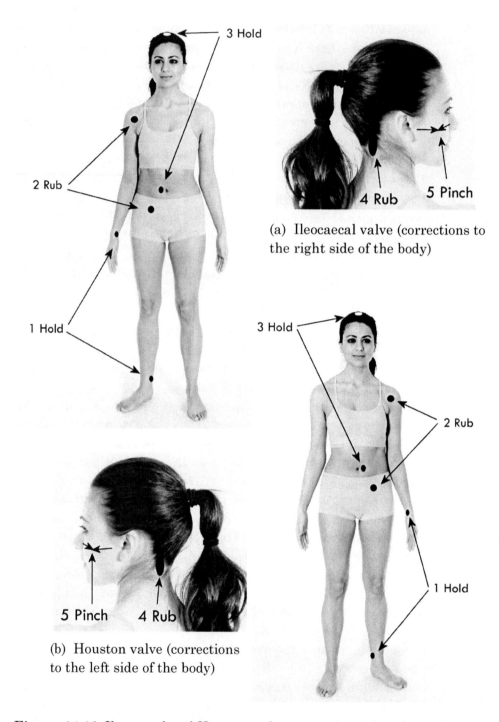

3 Hold

2 Rub

1 Hold

4 Rub   5 Pinch

(a) Ileocaecal valve (corrections to the right side of the body)

3 Hold

2 Rub

1 Hold

5 Pinch   4 Rub

(b) Houston valve (corrections to the left side of the body)

Figure 14.12 Ileocaecal and Houston valve correction points for under-energy

(vi)   Massage just to the side of the third cervical, near the top of the back of the neck (20 seconds).

(vii)   Pinch the zygomatic arch (the smile reflexes on the face) three times.

(viii) Put your feet together or tap your brow (to take the under-energized meridian out of circuit).

(ix)   Re-test the meridian by touching the kidney alarm point with heavy pressure. It should now be clear.

5☐ Put both hands over the ileocaecal or Houston point and put your legs apart to put the point in circuit.

6☐ Pick up your pendulum and deliberately swing the pendulum on the YES axis. It should now happily maintain that swing, indicating that there is no longer a problem. If there is a signal change, repeat the correction.   A§

On the next page you'll find a table which includes all the corrections in the book, according to category. Although so far you have only got to # 35, already you have an extensive repertoire of corrections to work with, and this should make your self-therapy highly effective. But you might not want to wait any longer to find out (in the next chapter) how the pendulum can make EFT an even more efficient tool.

Electrical

#	Electrical	TEST	CORRECTION
1	Auditory perception	66	66
2	Visual perception	68	69
3	Brain integration (cross-crawl)	78	78
4	Brain integration (cross-crawl) with eye movements	–	81
5	Tracing the lemniscate (vision)	–	82
6	Tracing the lemniscate (writing)	–	84
7	Gait reflexes	84	85
16	Tracing the meridian	–	163
17	Acupoints to tonify and sedate	–	164
18	Central & governing hook-up	–	171
19	Time of day balance	–	173
20	Balancing acupoints	–	174
21	Tracing a meridian backwards (for pain)	–	177
26	Body polarity	232	233
31	Cloacal energy	244	244

Emotional

#	Emotional	TEST	CORRECTION
8	Emotional stress release (ESR)	91	91
9	Frontal/Occipital holding	–	98
10	Emotional Distress Release (EDR)	–	99
11	Colour balance	–	101
12	Acknowledging the involved emotion	–	126
15	Neuro-vascular (NV) reflexes	161	161
33	Emotional rigidity	248	248
43a	Balancing with Bach remedies (categories)	–	305
43b	Balancing with Bach remedies (bottles)	–	306

Biochemical

#	Biochemical	TEST	CORRECTION
14	Neuro-lymphatic (NL) reflexes	154	157
29	Adrenal stress	237	238
32	RNA/DNA	245	246
37	Environmental allergies & sensitivities	–	274
38	Food compatibility	–	283
39	Identifying food issues	–	286
40a	Identifying nutritional *deficiencies*	–	290
40b	Identifying nutritional *excesses*	–	290
41	Storage, preparation & eating	–	291
42	Benefits/detriments of a supplement	–	300

Structural

#	Structural	TEST	CORRECTION
27	Common integrative area	233	234
28	Fixation	236	236
30	Constricted cranials	240	240
35	Ileocecal & Houston valve imbalance	251	252

Other methods

#	Other methods	TEST	CORRECTION
13	Identifying the antecedents of an issue	–	131
22	Working with life choices	–	186
23	Modelling a third-person perspective	–	186
24	Generating a support system	–	189
25	Giving the problem back (1)	–	197
34	Giving the problem back (2)	–	249
36	Applying EFT	–	264

Note:

Form the digital finger modes one at a time (page 223). An indicator change means that a correction from this category is required. Go down the list, using the correction numbers or stating the name of the correction to find the required correction.

Table 14.1 Tests & corrections according to finger-mode category (& other correction methods)

15
Emotional Freedom Techniques

Emotional Freedom Techniques (EFT) is a brilliant therapy for resolving problems, particularly when used in conjunction with the pendulum. It is one of the simplest and most effective therapies ever developed. Easy to learn and apply, it can't do any harm and can only do you good – it is a perfect therapy for self-application.[1]

The creation of Gary Craig, EFT was designed as a simpler and more effective version of Roger Callahan's Thought Field Therapy (TFT), which was the first of the new wave of energy therapies deriving from kinesiology.

Roger Callahan describes his discovery that marked the birth of Thought Field Therapy. He had been working with a client, Mary, for over a year using traditional psychotherapy techniques, without any real success. Mary had a severe phobia of water and couldn't bear even to look at the ocean or take a deep bath. At one point during treatment, while working in Callahan's garden within sight of a swimming pool, Mary mentioned that when she experienced or thought of water she had a feeling in the pit of her stomach. Callahan had done some training in kinesiology and was aware that the area underneath the eye was the first point of the stomach meridian. In a moment of inspiration – desperation, he reports[2] – Callahan asked Mary to tap underneath her eye while thinking of her fear of water. She tapped for two minutes and then declared that her fear was gone. She rushed to the pool and

---

1   For more information on EFT go to the official site: www.emofree.com.

2   Roger J. Callahan, with Richard Trubo, *Tapping the Healer Within: Using Thought Field Therapy to instantly conquer your fears, anxieties and emotional distress* (Contemporary Books, 2001), p. 8.

splashed her face with water. That evening Mary drove to the Californian coast and, not having learnt to swim, waded in the water.

Realizing that tapping meridian points could be a breakthrough in the treatment of phobias and other problems, Callahan developed a complex therapeutic system which involved tapping the ends of different meridians in particular sequences for specific ailments. He called these sequences *algorithms*.

One of Callahan's students, Gary Craig, wondered what would happen if, instead of tapping a particular sequence of acupoints for a particular problem, *he tapped the end points of all the meridians, in the same order, for any problem*. He found that this was just as effective as the algorithms. Indeed, Gary Craig argued, since you could apply this sequence to *any* problem (rather than the specified problems assigned to an algorithm), EFT has a far wider application than TFT.

Gary Craig called his system Emotional Freedom Techniques (EFT). A much simpler system than TFT, EFT can be used by anyone with the minimum of instruction. Craig, an engineer by training but a master at marketing, determined to share his creation with the world. Consequently, EFT is widely known and promulgated.

The EFT procedure essentially involves identifying the problem; acknowledging it; tapping acupoints (most of which are at the beginning or end of the meridian); and doing eye movements.

As you know from an earlier discussion, any problem relates to *feelings* (rather than simply thoughts) – it is feelings that make you do things you don't want to do or prevent you from doing things you want to do. *Thoughts*, on the other hand, belong in the realm of the conscious mind, and you can change them (although they are *influenced* by feelings). Feelings are involuntary; they belong in the realm of the body. You can admit or deny your feelings, but feelings do not derive from the conscious mind. By transforming the *feelings* related to the problem, the problem is resolved.

The more specific your target, the greater your chances of success with tapping. Feelings are very specific and this is another good reason why they are a good target. For EFT to be most effective, identify and acknowledge the *feelings* involved in the problem, and then tap the acupoints.

In EFT, points of the twelve primary meridians and the central and governing channels are tapped (figure 15.1, page 262). Tapping the end points of the meridians, as I see it, helps to open (or stimulate) the valves between the channels, and this gets the energy flowing. Problems are associated with blocked channels and stagnant energy; tapping the ends of the meridians gets energy moving, helping the problem to dissipate.

However, before the points are tapped, there is another essential element of the procedure. The emotion is acknowledged in what is called the *set-up phrase*, while a point on the chest, called the *sore spot*, is massaged. The points are then tapped. This is followed by eye movements.[3]

1 The set-up phrase

The set-up phrase is a fundamental element of the procedure (even though it isn't always necessary). There are three parts to the EFT set-up phrase: (1) the emotion; (2) the affirmation; and (3) the choice.[4]

First, get in touch with the somatic feelings connected with the problem and tune into them. Notice the emotion that goes with those feelings.[5] The first part of the set-up phrase is:

---

3   Gary Craig insists that what he calls the *nine gamut* – omitted in this description – is taught in EFT training approved by him. In other respects, my intention has been to present a version of EFT that Craig himself would recognize and approve of. Traditionally, between the tapping and the eye movements a procedure was included, borrowed from TFT, that involved counting and humming. It was designed to incorporate both sides of the brain (music activates the right side of the brain and maths the left). Many EFT practitioners now omit this part of the process. In my experience it isn't necessary and I haven't used it for years. Gary Craig doesn't seem to use it much either. If you want to try it, when you get to this part of the process, keep tapping the point between the ring and little finger (the 'gamut' point, since there are a gamut of things to do while you tap it) as you do the following: count to four; hum the first few bars of any tune (such as *Happy birthday to you*); then count to four again. Conclude with the eye movements.

4   The third part, the choice, is attributed to Patricia Harrington. It can be omitted when appropriate (when it's not yet clear what the goal would be, for example). Although Gary Craig doesn't seem to use it much, it's a very valuable addition to the process. Your body can help you overcome a problem more easily when it knows what you want instead – i.e. your *choice* or your goal.

5   For a discussion of the relationship of feelings and emotions see chapter 7.

Even though I feel [uncomfortable emotion] . . . (for example: *Even though I feel angry . . .*)

What you are doing here is acknowledging the emotion – which is of prime importance – and putting it on line. It's vital that you choose the words that are right for you. If you feel *hurt and distressed,* use those words; if you feel *mad as hell,* say so. Acknowledge your true feelings and, as far as possible – since emotions are sometimes hard to put into words – find the most apt expression for them. I'm sure I don't need to tell you this, but make sure you are acknowledging your feeling, not your prejudice. (*Don't* say, for example: *Even though I feel he's an idiot.* That's simply your prejudice – even if true. Acknowledge that you feel hurt, let down, rejected or whatever.)

Second, make the affirmation:

. . . I deeply and completely accept myself . . .

This might be difficult for you if you feel you don't accept yourself. But say it anyway – with feeling, *as if* you mean it. Accepting yourself is a prerequisite of health and happiness. Saying it often enough will help it to become true. The phrase itself can be modified. You might prefer: *I love and accept myself; I accept and forgive myself; I know I'm okay* (this is often more appropriate for children); and so on. You can even do EFT on not accepting yourself: *Even though I feel I reject myself,[6] I completely accept myself.*

Third, state what you would like instead of the uncomfortable emotion. What do you choose to be instead? You might for example say, *I choose to*

> . . . *be confident*
> . . . *be strong*
> . . . *put it behind me*
> . . . *know I'm lovable*
> . . . *be safe and secure in myself*
> . . . *be myself whatever other people think*
> . . . *be calm and relaxed*
> . . . *let it go*

---

6 Preferring, as far as possible, to use *positive terms;* that is, terms that aren't a negation. *I reject myself* is a positive term in this context. *I do not accept myself* would be a negation.

Or anything else. As you know, every issue involves both a problem and a goal. The first part of the set-up phrase acknowledges the problem; the third part states the goal. You acknowledge the problem and let your body know what you want instead.

It's helpful to use the word *feel* when referring to the problem, and to use the word *be* or *am* when referring to the goal. For example, *Even though I* feel *ugly . . . I choose to know that I* am *attractive.* This acknowledges that the problem is only a feeling; it enables a greater identification with the goal; and it gives the goal more power than the problem.

While saying the set-up phrase, massage the *sore spot* on the chest: rub it deeply using a slow, circular motion. Repeat the set-up phrase three times while massaging the sore spot.

The entire set-up phrase will be something like this:

> *Even though I feel [uncomfortable emotion], I completely accept myself, and choose to [be] [goal].* (For example: *Even though I feel angry, I completely accept myself, and choose to be calm*; or *Even though I feel really pissed off, I love and accept myself and choose to let it go.*)

Repeat this three times while massaging the sore spot.[7]

2 Tap the acupoints

Your body has now been alerted to the problem and informed of the goal. With the problem on line the acupoints for each meridian are now tapped (figure 15.1, page 262). The problem, in the form of a reminder phrase, is repeated to keep the body focused.

Use two fingers to tap each point firmly but gently about seven times (it makes no difference which side of the body you tap on, and it's fine to change sides during a tapping sequence; it's also fine to tap both sides at once, with both hands, if you want to). Each point only takes a few seconds to tap. If

---

7   Instead of massaging the sore spot, you can tap the karate-chop point, which is also effective and easier to explain when working with a group, for example.

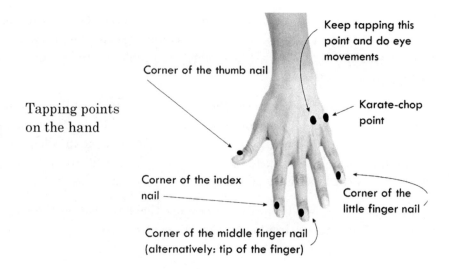

Tapping points
on the hand

Keep tapping this
point and do eye
movements

Corner of the thumb nail

Karate-chop
point

Corner of the index
nail

Corner of the
little finger nail

Corner of the middle finger nail
(alternatively: tip of the finger)

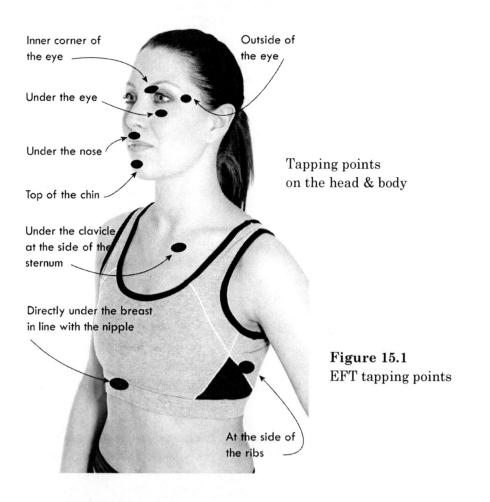

Inner corner of
the eye

Outside of
the eye

Under the eye

Under the nose

Top of the chin

Tapping points
on the head & body

Under the clavicle
at the side of the
sternum

Directly under the breast
in line with the nipple

At the side of
the ribs

Figure 15.1
EFT tapping points

the point feels tender, sensitive or painful, tap for longer (but maybe more gently; it's also okay to massage the point instead). As you tap, keep repeating the reminder phrase, *I feel* [uncomfortable emotion] (for example, *I feel angry*),[8] and stay with the feeling.

3 Eye rotation

As you tap the last of the points (between the ring finger and little finger on the back of the hand), look upwards and rotate your eyes clockwise, all the way round; take a breath; and rotate your eyes anticlockwise. If it helps, you can watch your fingers drawing circles in the air, keeping your head still, to help with the eye rotations (see figure 15.2) (you clearly can't keep tapping if you do this).[9] While you do the eye rotations, keep repeating the reminder phrase, stay with the feeling, and keep breathing.

It's time to put this into practice.

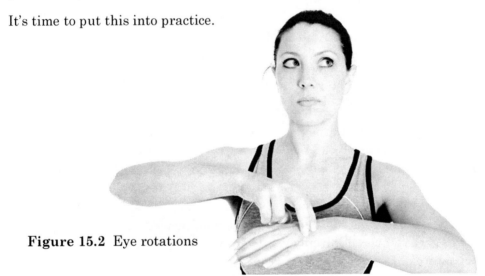

Figure 15.2 Eye rotations

---

8 People are sometimes concerned that they are repeating a negative affirmation. (This concern may be symptomatic of the pathological desire to avoid or deny uncomfortable emotions.) But this is *not* what you're doing. You are acknowledging the problem and holding it on-line so that you can balance your energies *in relation to the problem*. The idea is to resolve the problem, not just to bolster yourself.

9 There are a number of alternatives to eye rotations that may be equally helpful, such as looking sharply to the left and right and up and down; doing eye movements with eyes closed; and letting the eyes follow a sideways figure of eight (lemniscate) in the air.

36 CORRECTION
Applying EFT

1   Focus on something that makes you feel bad, or an issue.

2   Get in touch with the bad feeling and acknowledge the emotion. Take a SUD reading.

3   Decide how you would like to be instead. *Optional:* take a VOC reading.

4   Formulate the set-up phrase: *Even though I feel [uncomfortable emotion], I completely accept myself, and choose to [goal].*

5   Massage the sore spot and say the set-up phrase three times.

6   Tap the acupoints while repeating the reminder phrase, *I feel [uncomfortable emotion].*

7   Keep tapping the point between the ring finger and little finger, still repeating the reminder phrase, while you do the eye rotations (or follow two fingers on your hand with your gaze to help with the eye rotations).

8   Take a breath and relax. Notice what you feel now. Take a SUD reading. *Optional:* take a VOC reading of the goal.

After a round of tapping, reassess how you feel.

The SUD reading should have reduced and may now be at zero. If it isn't, check that the feelings you are measuring relate to the same target, and that the feelings you are measuring are the same ones you tapped on. Very often, when one target feeling is alleviated another, different feeling immediately presents itself. When this happens, you may feel just as bad, *but the feeling is a different one.* This is a sign that you're making progress. (In therapy, any change is good, even if initially you feel worse.) If the target changes, devise your set-up phrase for your new target and keep tapping.

If the original target is still giving you a negative SUD reading try re-tapping all the points. This may reduce your score further. If it makes no difference, you probably need to identify the source of the problem. However, EFT will usually instantly alleviate any problem, at least to some degree.

You can use the pendulum to find out which points to tap, but it's probably quicker and easier just to tap them all. Once you become practised in using EFT you can use your intuition to determine the points to tap. Tapping selectively quickens the process, which is obviously useful, but it doesn't make the tapping more effective.

If you find that EFT isn't working when really there's no reason why it shouldn't, Gary Craig suggests expressing the set-up phrase and reminder phrase loudly, with animation. My guess is that this helps to take the body out of fight or flight where it is in self-protection mode and restores it to a state receptive to help.[10] It's also possible that speaking loudly helps to keep focused and undistracted.

An alternative to saying the set-up phrase loudly is to do a few minutes of F/O holding while staying with the issue. Once your body is in a receptive state, try EFT again. It may be effective this time.

Some people respond exceptionally well to EFT. However, it does appear that with a few people EFT doesn't seem to help. But usually – actually, nearly always – when EFT doesn't seem to be working it is because the manifestations being tapped on are being held in place by deeper and more fundamental issues. These hidden sources have to be addressed first. The pendulum can help you to find them.

Aspects

If you tap on a problem in the present you are working with the *present manifestation* of a problem. You may resolve that particular manifestation, but there are other manifestations – other *aspects* – of the problem which may emerge at other times. For example, you feel awkward or inhibited in social situations. You tap on a social meeting in a bar with your work colleagues. Now it feels fine to be with your work colleagues socially in a bar. But the moment you walk into a bar with anyone you don't work with, the feelings resurface. And the bad feelings are not restricted to bars.

In EFT these different manifestations of a problem are referred to as *aspects*. The EFT literature encourages the explorer to tap on the various aspects of a

---

10   In EFT literature the collarbone breathing technique serves a similar function (in my estimation). The collarbone breathing technique is not outlined here since you already have techniques to deal with the fight/flight response, including ESR or F/O holding.

problem. The aspects are compared to trees in a forest. Each tree represents a different aspect. Keep chopping and you'll pretty soon have a clearing. With persistence all the trees in the forest will be felled. You probably won't need to attack every tree, since there is a generalization (domino) effect.

However, before you sharpen your metaphysical axe to get to work on the trees, there's a more simple and economical way. If, instead of tackling various manifestations of a problem in the present, you find the *sources* of the problem and resolve them, the problems in the present will no longer exist. Time travel, you see, is possible. Change the past and the present will be transformed. Unearthing the original seeds is far easier than felling the mature forest.

But how can you change what has happened in the past? What's done is done – isn't it? No. Not with regard to the traumas inhabiting your body. The past exists only as a representation in your body; that is all. It is a figment of your memory. It was real when it happened, but has no real existence in the present; it is only a representation. By changing that representation, all the manifestations change. It really is that simple.

Instead of applying EFT to the present manifestations of a problem, apply it to the source(s) of the problem. Once the sources are resolved, there will be no present manifestations – no aspects.[11]

Resolving the sources of the problem

Finding the sources of a problem – the *antecedent events* – is straightforward using the pendulum (see page 131, # 13: Identifying the antecedents of an issue). Exercise 15.1 shows you how to apply EFT to a problem's source.

Exercise 15.1 Resolving the source of a problem with EFT

1   Think of the problem you are going to work with. (Expect an indicator change as the pendulum registers this.)

---

11   Gary Craig insists that applying EFT successfully doesn't require identifying the sources of issues. But if you watch Gary in action, very often the tapping is ineffectual until, through persistence, the client reports the emergence of a memory. Once this memory (a source of the issue) is tapped on, the issue is able to be resolved.

2   Ask permission to work with this issue.

3   Determine what you would like instead of the problem. What is your goal?

4   Imagine being in the problem situation so that you can get in touch with the somatic feelings that are associated with the problem. Tune in to the feelings and acknowledge the involved emotions.

5   Ask if you need any more information in the present. If so, find out what.

6   Ask permission to go back in time to the sources of the problem. If you don't have permission, find out why and what you have to do first.[12]

7   Use the pendulum to take you back in time. Jump back in steps of five or ten years. When you get an indicator change, find the exact year. Bear in mind that it's possible that the issue involves a period of time which may be several years.

8   Direct your attention to what you were doing and what was happening during this time. Trust anything that pops into your head – but don't think about it (allow your unconscious body to communicate with you). Ask the pendulum to confirm you have found the right incident or relationship.

9   Identify the most effective target for EFT. You can get confirmation from the pendulum. Address the feelings.

10   Apply EFT.

11   Check if there is any more to be done at this time. If so, find out what and apply EFT to the problem.

12   Ask permission to return to the present. If granted, ask the pendulum to give you a signal change when you're back in the present.

13   Check if there are any other times in the past which you need to visit. If so, go to that time and proceed from point 8 above.

14   When you are back in the present, with no further corrections to make, check how you are feeling.

15   In your imagination visit various scenarios in the future which would have been a problem in the past. Notice how you feel in those situations now.

Your problem may now be completely resolved, or you may need to visit it again later and do some more work. The wonderful thing about going back

---

12   It is normally preferable to resolve an issue as far as possible in the present before going back in time.

into the past and resolving the problem at the source is that it is then gone
for good. You won't be able to get the problem back. Of course, resolving the
present problem may require a number of sessions, depending on the number
of antecedent events; and it may take more than one session to resolve any
particular trauma.

You can do exercise 15.1 using all the corrections you've learned, not just
EFT. Ask, *Is EFT the most useful correction?* If it isn't, find out what is.

I shouldn't leave a discussion of EFT without mentioning what's called
psychological reversal. Psychological reversal is the term that's often used
to explain when EFT 'doesn't work'. The notion is that, if EFT isn't working,
this is because the energy flow in the channels is somehow 'reversed'.

This is a misconception. It is easy to see how it comes about. Imagine, for example, that you have a fear of water. You've tried EFT on a present manifestation (or aspect) and it hasn't worked. You are then muscle tested. You are
asked to say, 'I want to get over my fear of water', and the indicator muscle
unlocks. This has been called 'psychological reversal' because you think you
want to get over your problem, but your body disagrees. The results of the
test is reversed: instead of a locked response (meaning, yes, I want to get over
my fear of water), you get an unlocked response (meaning, no, I don't want
to get over this fear). The perceived reversal of response is erroneously interpreted to mean there is a reversal of energy flow; that energy is somehow
flowing backwards. This is decidedly *not* what is happening.

In fact, the formulation 'I want to get over my problem' is unfortunate. A
kinesiologist (most EFT practitioners are not kinesiologists) would usually
expect an unlocking muscle in response to this statement, because putting on
line the fear of water is a stress to the body (even if, on every level, the person
does want to get over the problem).

If EFT isn't working, it isn't due to 'psychological reversal' or energy flowing
the wrong way (which would be exceedingly rare and possibly fatal), but is
likely to be because there are traumas and connected beliefs that need to
be processed first. Consciously, you may want to get over a fear of water;
unconsciously, the body may believe (as a result of specific experience) that
water is dangerous – hence the fear.

You can test yourself, using the pendulum, to uncover any unconscious beliefs which are maintaining the problem. Use +/– mode and make statements

to find out whether your body agrees with them. Here are examples of such statements:

- I want to get over this problem.
- I believe I can get over this problem.
- It is safe for me to get over this problem.
- It is safe for others for me to get over this problem.
- I will still be loved if I get over this problem.
- I will be happy if I get over this problem.

If any of these statements give you a NO/STRESSED, find out why. All unhelpful beliefs come from experiences or (less often) parental brainwashing.[13] If you have an unhelpful belief which your body is unwilling to let go of, it is highly likely that it derives from a traumatic experience in your past. Use the pendulum to identify the experience, and use EFT (and other kinesiology methods) to resolve it. By resolving the trauma the belief will change automatically.

EFT is a highly effective therapeutic method. You can use it in the present to alleviate any symptom. When used in conjunction with the pendulum to resolve the sources of the problem, EFT becomes so much more effective.

You can use EFT along with other kinesiology methods as part of a balance; or you can use EFT exclusively as a quick way of clearing the sources of a problem. You don't even need a pendulum to do it: you can do EFT anywhere at any time. If you are embarrassed about tapping in public, tap on that issue; alternatively, surreptitiously hold the points and breathe. You can even tap in your imagination.

Anything can be helped with EFT. In addition to emotional issues, use EFT for any physical ailments. Use it when you feel unwell or when you feel illness coming on (be as specific as possible about your symptoms). If you have time, discover the underlying sources of the problem and give yourself a balance; if you have only five minutes, give yourself some EFT.

As Gary Craig says, try it on everything!

---

13   Or brainwashing performed by the primary carers, if these are not your parents.

16
Environmental Factors

There's a lot the pendulum can't tell you, such as the winning numbers or the weather next week. There's a lot it might be unwilling to tell you (at least until you have defused your stress in relation to it), such as whether your spouse is having an affair or what exactly happened when you were six.[1] And there's a lot you probably shouldn't be asking (such as whether there is a heaven), because the pendulum doesn't give you privileged access to classified information. As you may have already discovered, the pendulum will probably give you some answer to anything you ask. But the answer isn't necessarily true. A kinesiologist who declares otherwise I'd recommend avoiding.[2]

Self-responsibility

You certainly shouldn't ask the pendulum to make your personal decisions for you. You can ask the pendulum for information to help you to make an informed decision, but the decision itself is for your conscious mind to make. Don't attempt to abdicate responsibility by passing your decisions on to your unconscious. Taking decisions is your responsibility as a conscious being. We are all responsible for our actions; that is the bottom line. You are account-

---

1   And even if it does tell you, you can't assume that it is God's truth. These would be inappropriate uses of the pendulum, you might be disappointed to learn. Don't go there.

2   This issue is no different from the controversies of *false memory* in hypnosis, where evangelical hypnotists have encouraged people to make false accusations (usually of child sexual abuse) after 'recovering' (actually, *creating*) false memories through hypnosis. Hypnosis gives no privileged access to God's Truth; and neither does kinesiology.

able. Moral responsibility, whether we like it or not, is the human condition. It comes automatically with consciousness. It's written on the box.[3]

However, there's a lot of useful information you can get from your unconscious body through the pendulum. As well as information about your emotional well-being and the best remedy, the pendulum can give you important information about how your environment is affecting you.

Children

If you have children, using yourself as a surrogate, the pendulum can also give you very useful information about how the environment is affecting them too (regarding surrogacy, see chapter 3).

Children are generally much more sensitive than adults. As far as you can – but I'm sure you don't need me to tell you this – serve up food that is fresh (unprocessed) and preferably organic (and therefore free from harmful additives and preservatives), including plenty of *tasty* fruit and vegetables (trying to make children eat tasteless or unpleasant fruit or vegetables on the grounds that it's good for them will just put them off). Create an environment that is, as far as possible, clear of stressors and poisons. This will help your children to remain free of the illnesses and ailments (such as asthma, eczema and allergies) associated with environmental toxins, and give them more resilience to cope with such toxins when they can't avoid them.

Environmental stressors

Environmental stressors can be as severe as emotional stressors for some people. If you have suffered a great deal of emotional stress your tolerance of harmful environmental stimuli is likely to be reduced, and vice-versa. There does seem to be a constitutional (genetic) factor regarding the degree of toxic stimuli a human body can tolerate.

Environmental stressors can relate directly to a particular experience or trauma from the past. Allergies and sensitivities – whether to benign or toxic substances – often arise as a result of a trauma. They also commonly arise

---

3   For a discussion of this, see chapter 6.

as a result of repeated or extended exposure to a particular substance. This applies to foods as well. People are commonly sensitive to foods they eat too much of.

The pendulum will tell you whether a substance you are sensitive to can be rendered tolerable or whether you need to do your best to avoid it. But exercise caution with such communications: your body doesn't necessarily know now what it will be able to cope with in a month or two. You may need to ask at regular intervals.

Warning:

If you have a severe allergic reaction to any substance *do not* imagine coming into contact with it, because of the risk of anaphylaxis. Even summoning up an allergen in your imagination can trigger an allergic response. Treatment of severe allergies should only be undertaken in the presence of a medical doctor. There is a risk of anaphylactic shock.

Use the pendulum to find out which substances you are sensitive to. You can do this in your imagination as well as by introducing the actual substance. Simply imagine coming into contact with the substance in whatever context you experience the reaction (e.g. smelling it; seeing it). Once you have identified the substance (e.g. grass pollen, dust, fur), ask the pendulum if there's anything you can do to help. Almost certainly you will be able to help – even if you can't completely resolve it. Carry out a full balance on a goal such as: My *body is relaxed and comfortable in the presence of* X. If you take a pendulum SUD reading before and after the balance, you will know how much you've achieved.

To identify a substance you are sensitive or allergic to, use the pendulum in +/– mode. If the pendulum changes its swing to NO–STRESSED when you introduce the substance (in actuality or in your imagination), the substance is stressful to the body. This is a similar principle to muscle testing in kinesiology, where an unlocking muscle would represent stress. But whereas in kinesiology the unlocking muscle is (perhaps) purely a physiological reaction to stress, the change of swing of the pendulum is a deliberate communication by the unconscious.

Allergies to harmless substances are very often straightforward to eliminate. Allergies or sensitivities to toxic or harmful substances (and sometimes to foods – see chapter 17), on the other hand, can be more difficult to resolve and it may not be possible to resolve them completely. It's not always possible to determine whether a substance you are sensitive to is actually harmful or benign, since we are all constituted differently – one person's meat being another's poison. The body certainly responds to such substances as if they are harmful.

The procedure to overcome environmental allergies or sensitivities (method # 37)[4] is most likely to be effective with benign environmental allergies (such as cat hair or pollen). It might not be successful with food allergies or toxic substances such as household chemicals (which may not be an immune system *mistake*). However, even toxic household substances your body should be able to tolerate in small enough quantities (but if your body has been subject to too many toxins over a period of time it may require a complete break for some while).

37 CORRECTION
Environmental allergies and sensitivities

Warning: don't do this exercise if there is a risk of anaphylactic shock without the supervision of a medical doctor who is physically present.

1☐   Do the pre-checks.
2☐   Ask: *Do I have permission to work with this allergy/sensitivity right now?* (If you don't have permission, don't even think about it.)
3☐   Bring to mind the matter you're sensitive too, and watch the pendulum change from YES–POSITIVE to NO–STRESSED.
4☐   Ask your body if there are any *positive intentions* regarding your body being sensitive to the matter. In other words, is there anything positive or useful your body wants to achieve from having this sensitivity?[5] If so:
      (i)   Find out what the positive intention is. (Just ask, and let your unconscious body tell you – don't *think* about it; just tune into

---

4   Adapted from Connirae and Steve Andreas, *Heart of the Mind* (Real People Press, 1989), pages 37 forward.
5   A common positive intention is for *protection*.

your body and let it tell you through an intuition – and confirm the answer with the pendulum.)

(ii)   Ask permission first and then go back in time to find out where it comes from. It will almost certainly derive from an unprocessed trauma.

(iii) Elicit as much information your body says you need about the trauma.

(iv)   Resolve the trauma using any of the techniques you've learnt – letting your body tell you the optimum methods.

(v)   Return to the present.

5□ Ask your body if it's now ready to help you resolve the sensitivity or allergy. If it's not, do F/O holding or find what needs to be done first.

6□ Let your body know that very often an allergy or sensitivity is an error of the immune system, where something benign is mistaken for a harmful substance.

7□ Think of the substance you're sensitive to (let's call it an allergen for short) – *providing it's safe to do so*. Notice your physical reaction.

8□ Think of something similar to the matter you're sensitive to (or allergen) which your body has no problem with. (For example dog hair, if you're allergic only to cat hair.) Notice how your body responds appropriately (that is to say, neutrally).

9□ Imagine a glass screen in front of you, and on the other side, completely isolated from you, is a version of you (like an image or reflection of you) that has no such sensitivity.

10□ Watch this image of yourself, as the substance that presents no problem (such as the dog hair) is introduced to this other self. Then watch as the allergen (such as cat hair) is introduced. Notice how this version of yourself responds appropriately, accepting the substance as benign.

11□ Watch again, more carefully, and see how your other self is completely calm in the presence of the problem substance. And also note how your own body (this side of the screen) has no reaction while you watch yourself on the other side of the screen. Make sure both bodies are entirely comfortable. (If not, you need to backtrack, probably looking at positive intentions again.)

12□ Take down the imaginary glass screen and bring this other self back into your body. Invite this self to show you how to accept the formerly problem substance appropriately.

13□ Then imagine the substance that was previously an allergen being introduced to you. Notice how your body accepts it calmly and easily.

14□ Thank your body for its help. Imagine yourself in future situations in the presence of the substance, noticing how comfortable your body feels.

Cell phones

There are many substances in the environment that are detrimental to everyone, not because an individual is 'sensitive' to them (the term implies an individual predisposition), but because they deplete human energy.

The cell phone test (exercise 16.1) will almost certainly produce a stress response caused by the electromagnetic waves. You won't need any persuasion of the ill effects of cell phones if, like many people, you experience head pains when you hold the handset close to your head for any length of time. Avoid using the cell phone more than you have to; or use a speakerphone facility so it's not so close to the head.

Exercise 16.1 Cell phone sensitivity

1☐   Have the pendulum swinging on the YES–POSITIVE axis.
2☐   Bring your (turned on) cell phone to your ear. A signal change means your body is negatively affected by the presence of the phone.

Synthetic materials

Many people are stressed by wearing synthetic materials. Check your sports clothes, which are usually made of synthetic materials. Do this by having the pendulum swinging on the YES–POSITIVE axis, and then hold the garment in your hand or hold it against your skin. If the pendulum swings to the NO–STRESSED axis you know that the garment stresses your body. Test your hats by putting them on and noticing what happens to the pendulum.

If you want to test a garment that you are wearing, have the pendulum swinging on the YES–POSITIVE axis and touch the *inside* of the garment. Notice whether the pendulum gives a signal change. Test your underwear in this way. Women in particular are likely to wear synthetic underwear. If you wear an underwire bra, see if it stresses you.

If your sheets are not 100 per cent cotton, check them in the same way as your clothes.

Chemicals

You may be sensitive to any of the minefield of chemicals many people have in their homes.

Check your deodorant. If it's also an anti-perspirant it probably contains aluminium which the body absorbs and may be linked with Alzheimer's. If your body is familiar with it, you needn't actually apply it. With the pendulum swinging on the YES–POSITIVE axis, just pick the deoderant up with your other hand and imagine applying it. If the pendulum changes its swing you know that the product stresses your body.

Do the same with your other cosmetics: your soap, shampoo, toothpaste, face cleanser, moisturizers, perfumes and so on. Again, providing your body is familiar with them, there is no need to apply them. Hold them in your hand and imagine applying them. Do you really want to use products on a daily basis which stress your body? The body is versatile, accommodating and very forgiving, but these stresses are cumulative. You probably can't do much to avoid vehicle fumes, but there are plenty of other stressors you can easily eliminate. Some people are of course more sensitive than others to environmental pollutants. The finer your hair and skin, the more sensitive you're likely to be. Very few skin-care product ranges are completely natural and non-toxic. Use your pendulum to find the best for you. Dr.Hauschka skincare products, for example, based on organic and biodynamically grown ingredients, are free from any synthetic or toxic substances.

Test your detergent by touching or smelling your clothes when they come out of the washing machine. If the pendulum changes to NO–STRESSED, you may want to find a more natural detergent.

You might also want to test your household cleaning materials – especially if you have babies or young children. The increase in asthma, eczema and allergies among children is almost certainly related to the toxic chemicals (and bad food) many are exposed to daily. You can test whether your children or other family members are sensitive to any product by using yourself as a surrogate (see chapter 3).

If you use chemicals in your work, test your response to them as well.

Electro-magnetic radiation

As well as cell phones, there are a number of other common sources of electro-magnetic radiation. Computers, television, and florescent lighting can stress the body.

Of course, you can't simply completely eliminate all the environmental stressors – just as you can't eliminate all the emotional stressors. Use the table to record the degree of stress by taking a reading, where 100 represents extreme stress and zero means none at all. You can work in general categories or identify the stress of specific items. You needn't take a reading of every stressor; find the priorities.

Ask whether there is anything you can do to reduce the stress (through balancing yourself or avoiding the stressor) and record this under *Action*. You are also invited to use the pendulum to establish an overall reading of environmental stress and compare it to your overall emotional stress. The results can be enlightening.

	Date	Stress / 100	Action	Date	Stress / 100	Action
Cosmetics						
Detergents						
Computer						
TV						
Cell phone						
Other (find what)						
Overall home						
Overall work						
Outside						
Total environ-mental stressors						
Total emotional stressors						

Table 16.1 Environmental stress

The healthier and more balanced you are, the greater your resources in dealing with environmental and other stressors. Keep yourself balanced with kinesiology techniques to raise your tolerance levels.

Geopathic stress & feng shui

Geopathic stress relates to earth energies that have a deleterious effect on the energies of the body. Equally, features of the environment itself can enhance or adversely affect the body's energies – this is the realm of feng shui. A discussion of these two fields is beyond the scope of this book – and my expertise. However, it may be very helpful to use the pendulum to read the energetic topography of your home and workspace and find ways to improve them.

How well do you sleep at night? As we noted earlier (chapter 11), quality of sleep is a key general indicator of stress. One of the stressors might be the positioning of your bed or which way round you sleep. Ask the pendulum if your bed is in the best location for optimum sleep. You can always record a percentage, where 100 per cent is the best location for optimum sleep and zero means sleep is impossible. Ask the pendulum if there are other locations in the bedroom that would be better. Take a percentage reading for here too. It might improve your sleep if you take a different room as your bedroom (supposing this to be possible).

But it might not be the location of your bed *per se* but the location of – for example – the television directly in line with it in the room below or above. Or it may be that a mirror is pointing directly at the bed and simply moving the mirror (or covering it at night) would render the bed location perfect. Ask the pendulum if there is a solution other than moving the bed. Find out what else you can do.

The chances are that moving your bed will upset the aesthetics of the room. If there's only a few percentage points difference it may not be worth it, but if your sleep currently is terrible and a different location would transform the quality of your sleep, it may be worth the effort or inconvenience.

You can do similar work with any other part of your house or office. Check if your desk is in the right position, and whether you are facing in the right direction. Again, take a percentage reading. It may be that by moving the

desk, changing its angle, or altering the position of your chair you can become more productive in your work.

You might consider getting a book on geopathic stress or feng shui and consulting it in collaboration with the pendulum. The pendulum can help you
to make priorities about what to change, and also how to harmonize your
environment using crystals, mirrors, pictures and other artefacts, if you're
into that kind of thing.

17
Food & Nutrition

How good is your diet? Even if it's very good, are the foods that you eat the best for your body? Are you getting the nutrition you need to function optimally? Do you need a particular diet to help you achieve your sporting goals or to make it easy to become slim? Are you sensitive to some of the foods that you eat? Are there other factors – which you may not even be aware of – relating to your eating that aren't serving you as well as possible?

The pendulum can help you to identify:

- The best foods for you at any particular time.
- The best diet for your body.
- The 'good' foods that aren't good for your individual body at this time.
- The specific diet that can help you achieve a goal.
- Your nutritional needs in relation to a specific problem.
- The foods or nutrients that will help to balance your body.
- The nutrients that you are deficient in.
- Food sensitivities and allergies.
- Foods you should avoid or eat less of.
- Which foods increase or decrease your energy levels.
- Other factors to help you to digest and get the nutrients from your food.

Clearly, the more you know about nutrition, the more the pendulum can help you with your diet. At the very least, the pendulum can help you to identify foods you should or shouldn't be eating. If you need professional assistance, see a kinesiologist who specializes in nutrition; or a nutritionist competent in the use of muscle testing.

If you are the parent of young children with behavioural problems, do you suspect that their behaviour is influenced by the food they're eating? With yourself as surrogate (see chapter 3) you can use the pendulum to identify the best foods for your children and the foods that are harming them. Children who are hyperactive or unable to give sustained attention to an activity may well be eating foods that are harmful.[1]

Optimizing your diet can help you to:

- Increase energy
- Achieve your ideal weight
- Guard against illness
- Generate positive moods and stabilize blood-sugar levels
- Stimulate libido
- Improve athletic performance
- Sleep well
- Improve physical appearance
- Maintain good health

Generally speaking – for an optimum diet adhere to the following guidelines:[2]

- Eat plenty of fresh fruit and vegetables.[3]
- Drink plenty of pure water.
- Eat food that is organic (biodynamic if available).
- Eat fresh sea fish.
- Only use sea salt (not table salt).
- Avoid processed foods – the more processed a food, the more you should avoid it. This way you avoid food devested of nutrients; food invested with additives; food containing vast quantities of salt,

---

1   Foods that contain additives, for example, may be poisonous to the child, who then needs to keep active in order to expel the toxins from the body as quickly as possible. Or the child may be sensitive or allergic to certain foods or substances in foods.

2   For more information see Patrick Holford, *Optimum Nutrition Bible* (Piatkus Books, 2004).

3   'The Government recommends an intake of at least five portions of fruit or vegetables per person per day to help reduce the risk of some cancers, heart disease and many other chronic conditions' (British Department of Health). Research by Professor Gerry Potter of De Montfort University, Leicester, has discovered that a class of molecules called *salvestrols* have significant anti-cancer and other healing benefits. Salvestrols are naturally found in the skin of fruits and vegetables, but are absent when these are sprayed with synthetic fungicides. For the research, go to www.naturesdefence.com. A supplement is available through www.fruitforce.co.uk.

fat and refined sugar; and food that doesn't even look or taste like food.

○ Eat red meat in moderation.

○ When using oil in cooking, use groundnut (peanut) oil or olive oil (to avoid trans-fatty acids).

○ Eat butter not margarine (because of the trans-fatty acids produced when vegetable oils are hardened artificially).

○ Avoid refined sugar.

○ Avoid 'diet' drinks, particularly those containing aspartame.

○ Consume in moderation foods high in fat or cholesterol.

○ Eat food that is in season.

○ Eat wheat (including bread) only in moderation.

○ Drink alcohol only in moderation.

○ Avoid chemically decaffeinated coffee and consume coffee only in moderation.

Use the pendulum to determine what constitutes moderation for you. Remember that your results will depend on your frame of reference. A possible frame of reference (the one I use for myself) is: *the amount of coffee (for example) that will allow me to live a healthy life to age one hundred.*

Testing foods

Testing foods is very straightforward (# 38). There are four possibilities: the food is good for you (*biogenic*); detrimental to you (*biocidic*); neither good nor bad (*biostatic*); or both good and bad (*biogenic* and *biocidic*). If a food is both biogenic and biocidic there are nutrients in the food the body needs, but there is something about the food that is detrimental. Don't forget to do all the necessary pre-checks and to ask permission.

38 CORRECTION
Testing food compatibility

1 Bring the food close to your body. You can place it next to your navel or your cheek (the parotid gland on the side of your jaw).

2 If you get an indicator change, the food has some effect on your energy system.

3   Apply palm mode and ask: *Is this food beneficial to me?* An indicator change suggests it is beneficial (biogenic).

4   Apply palm mode and ask: *Is this food detrimental to me?* An indicator change suggests it is detrimental (biocidic).

5   If you get no indicator change for either question, the food is neither good nor bad (biostatic).

If you get an indicator change for both points 3 and 4, there are nutrients in the food that you need, but the food also contains something detrimental. There are a number of things you can do.

1   Apply priority mode. If you get an indicator change your body is saying that consuming this food is a priority.

2   Identify an alternative food that provides the nutrients the body needs but is not detrimental.

3   Apply totality mode from the next chapter (figure 18.1, page 301). A signal change means that, overall, the food is more beneficial than detrimental.

Even more reliable than putting the food close to the body (# 38, point 1) is to put it in the mouth and briefly chew (but don't swallow). The pendulum will tell you if the food is beneficial or not. Putting a food in your mouth is *not* a good idea if you are sensitive or allergic to it. (If you don't have the food to hand, you can simply *imagine* that you are eating it, and test with the pendulum.)

Then imagine you have eaten the food and it is digesting. Test again. Some foods show up as detrimental only in the process of digesting, rather than eating.

If in doubt, before eating any meal or snack, check that the food will nourish you and not harm you. This can prove an expensive – or unpopular – activity in restaurants, cafés and fast-food outlets, but it could improve your health.

You can balance yourself specifically for food and nutrition; or you can include nutrition as part of a general balance. The latter involves including foods and nutrients among the corrections as you follow the general protocol. The finger mode for nutrition is thumb pad to middle finger pad (figure 17.1).

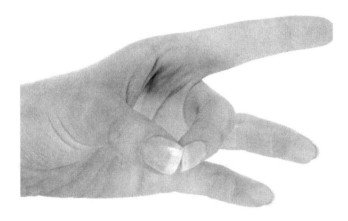

Figure 17.1 Nutrition/biochemical finger mode

Balancing specifically for foods and nutrition

You can make a conscious choice about the dietary issues to address, and use the pendulum to determine the nature of the issue and the best resolution.

Alternatively, you can ask your body to determine the issue. Ask: *Is there an issue relating to eating and nutrition that would be useful to address now?* If there is, find out whether the issue relates to:

1☐ Foods (including water and other drinks).
2☐ Nutrients.
3☐ Storage, preparation and eating.

The sections that follow will help you to explore these areas in detail.

Foods

This area includes drinks and oils, and anything else you might put into your stomach.

Where you need to identify a specific food, decide (or ask the pendulum) which category to use. Then use the pendulum to narrow it down to the specific food. (The culinary groups and nutritional groups tables are at the end of this chapter.)

- ○ Culinary groups (table 17.2, pages 292–5).
- ○ Nutritional groups (table 17.3, page 295).
- ○ Ridler's reflexes (figure 17.2, pages 288–9).

Bear in mind that it is possible that your body wants to refer to a whole group rather than a particular food.

Method # 39 will help you to identify issues with foods. You will identify whether the issue concerns *quality* or *quantity*. Then take the appropriate steps: eat less (or none) or more of the food, or remedy the quality.

39 CORRECTION
Identifying food issues

Quantity

1   Ask: *Is there an issue with the* quantity *of food I'm eating?* If the answer is NO go to point 5.
2   If so, ask: *Am I consuming too much of a food?* Also ask: *Am I consuming too little of a food?*
3   Ask the pendulum which category to use to determine the food or nutrient you're eating too little or too much of (culinary group; nutritional group; Ridler reflexes). Use that category to identify the specific food (or group of foods). Alternatively, or in addition, use your intuition, and check with the pendulum.
4   Once you have identified the food, find out how much you should (or shouldn't) be eating. Some foods you may need to avoid altogether, at least for a while. Also check that you are drinking enough (pure) water.

Quality

5   Ask: *Is there an issue with the* quality *of food I am eating?* If so, find out what the issue is. For example, are you eating enough *fresh* foods; should you be eating more *organic* food? Check that you have established everything your body wants you to do.

6   Ask: *Is there anything else I need to know?* If so, find out what.

7   Finally, find out when you should test again. Things may be different tomorrow, next week or next month.

Tip:

When working with the pendulum, use your intuition, and always trust any ideas that pop up in your head.

Nutrients

If the issue is nutrients, use the Ridler reflexes (figure 17.2, page 288) to identify the nutritional deficiency (or excess). When you use the Ridler chart to locate the nutrients required, you can point to the points on the chart itself or touch your own body. Pointing to the chart is quicker than finding the point on the body; but to ensure accuracy I suggest that, after an excess or deficiency has been indicated on the chart, you then double-check by touching the relevant point on your body.

You can use the Ridler points as part of a balance or on their own to identify nutritional needs without reference to any particular problem or goal.

Be clear in your own mind whether you are testing for excesses or deficiencies. If unsure, you can say: G*ive me an indicator change if this is a deficiency.*

Warning:

Toxic chemicals and heavy metals should only come up as an excess, *never* as a deficiency.

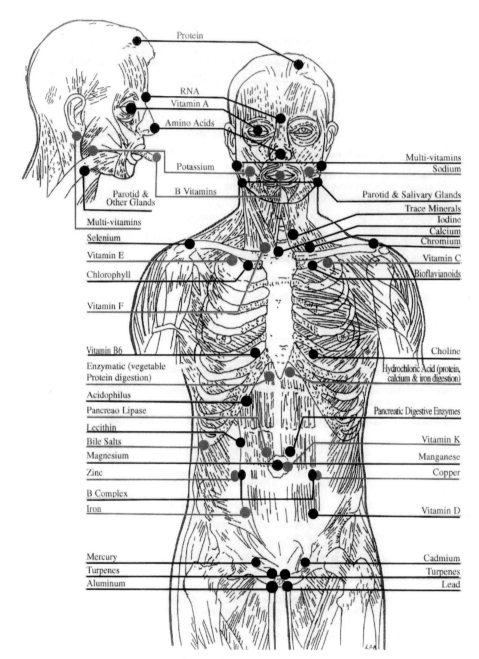

Figure 17.2 Ridler reflex points

Source: Based on Dr Ridler's research, this chart includes later modifications and additions, compiled by Dr Charles Krebs. Reproduced with kind permission.

Notes on figure 17.2: Nutritional labels according to category and how to locate on the body

Vitamins

Vitamin A
 Centre of eyelid of right eye
B vitamins
 Tip of tongue
B complex
Choline
Vitamin B6
Vitamin C
Vitamin D
Vitamin E
Vitamin F
Vitamin K

Multivitamins:
 Just under the ear where the lobe joins the face. It is suggested that both sides of the face should be touched at the same time. Do this, and bring your legs together and apart, to lock in circuit. Begin to swing the pendulum on the YES/ POSITIVE axis. If it immediately changes to the NO/NEGATIVE axis, multivitamins are indicated
Bioflavanoids

Minerals

Calcium
Copper
Chromium
Iodine
Iron
Magnesium

Manganese
Potassium
Selenium
Sodium
Trace minerals

Proteins & enzymes

Amino acids
Enzymatic (vegetable protein
 digestion)

Parotid & salivary amylase

Other nutrients

Acidophilus
Bile salts
Chlorophyll
Hydrochloric acid
Lecithin

RNA
Pancreaolipase pancreatic
Digestive enzymes
Protein
 Touch the hair

Toxic chemicals & heavy metals
(Should appear only as excess)

Aluminium
Cadmium
Lead

Mercury
Turpenes

40a CORRECTION
Identifying nutritional *deficiencies*

1   After the usual pre-checks and when permission is granted, ask: *Do I have any nutritional deficiencies?*
2   If you do, put this into circuit by putting your legs apart as the pendulum produces a signal change. Keep this mode in circuit till the end of the exercise.
3   With your fingers or hand, cover the head area on the Ridler chart. Be clear in your own mind which points you are including.
4   If you get an indicator change, find out which reflexes have indicated. Narrow it down by covering a group of the reflexes, or point to each in turn, until you have the nutritional deficiencies from this area.
5   Double check by neutral touching the corresponding point on your own body. The same points should indicate.
6   With your fingers or hand, cover the chest area of the chart. Repeat points 4 and 5 above.
7   Cover the abdomen area and repeat points 4 and 5.
8   Once you have all the deficiencies, if appropriate, find the priorities. Retest the indicated nutrients (on your body) with priority mode and using two fingers for a neutral touch. Any that produce an indicator change are a priority.
9   Terminate the circuit.

40b CORRECTION
Identifying nutritional *excesses*

To test for nutritional excesses, repeat # 40a, replacing the question in number 1 to: Do I have any nutritional excesses? *If you get an indicator change, put it into circuit. Now anything that shows up will be an excess. Heavy metals, which are to be avoided completely, may show up as an excess.*

Storage, preparation and eating

If the issue is not about food itself but rather food storage, preparation or eating, the following method will identify the problem.

41 CORRECTION
Storage, preparation and eating

1   Ask: *Are there issues with the storage, preparation or eating of food?*
2   If so, one or more of the following will indicate (if more than one, find
      the priority – or have the intention that just one will indicate): *Storage.*
      Preparation. Eating. Go to the relevant column of table 17.1.
3   Identify the subcategory.
4   Establish the issue as precisely as possible. Use your intuition and
      keep asking *Do I need any more information?* until you have all the
      information you need.
5   Determine the most appropriate and efficient action to resolve the
      issue, checking with the pendulum.
6   Go to number 1 above, and repeat with any further issues.

Storage	Preparation	Eating
Age/time	Food Combining (e.g. Hay	Posture
Cooking utensils	diet)[1]	Ritual
Freshness	Method of cooking (e.g.	Environment
Packaging	frying, microwave)	Times
Storage place	Raw foods	Chewing & speed
Temperature	Under/overcooking	Quantity
Other	Utensils	Attention-conscious
	Other	eating
		Drinking while eating
		Other

Table 17.1 Storage, preparation, eating

Source: Adapted from Jane Thurnell-Read, Nutrition Session Menu, in
Nutrition for Kinesiologists (course manual, 2003).

---

1   The Hay diet recommends that carbohydrates are not eaten with proteins.
This is because proteins require an acid medium for digestion while carbohydrates require an alkaline medium. When eaten together the stomach is unable to digest either food properly. Vegetables can be eaten with either proteins
or carbohydrates. Fruit should be eaten separately – well before or well after a
meal of protein or carbohydrate.

CHICKEN

MEAT

> *Identify the type of meat*

FISH

> *Identify the type of fish*

DAIRY & EGG

      butter
      cream
      milk
      eggs

FRUIT

berries

blackberry	currant
blueberry	gooseberry
cranberry	raspberry
	strawberry
	other

citrus

citron	lime
grapefruit	mandarin (tangerine)
kumquat	orange
lemon	

apple	guava	peach	quince
apricot	mango	pear	rhubarb
banana	melon	persimmon	*other exotic fruit*
cherry	nectarine	pineapple	
date	olive	plantain	
fig	papaya	plum	
grape	passion fruit	pomegranate	

Table 17.2 Culinary groups (*continues*)

Table 17.2 *(cont'd)*

VEGETABLES

bulbs

chive
garlic
leek
onion
shallot

cabbages

broccoli
Brussel sprout
cabbage
cauliflower
turnip
other

gourds

chayote
cucumber
pumpkin
squash
other

leafy greens

chard	lettuce
chicory	mustard
cress	rocket
dan delion	sorrel
kale	spinach

legumes

beans

black-eyed bean/pea	lima bean
haricot bean	mung bean
kidney bean	pinto bean
runner bean	*other*
string bean	

pea
chickpea
lentil
peanut
soy bean
other

nightshades

egg plant (aubergine)
pepper
tomato

root vegetables

arrowroot	malanga
artichoke	parsnip
beet	potato
carrot	radish
cassava	sweet potato
horseradish	yam

Table 17.2 *(cont'd)*

MUSHROOMS

SEEDS

    grains

barley	rice
buckwheat	rye
corn	wheat
millet	*other*
oats	

    nuts

almond	macadamia
beech nut	pecan
brazil nut	pine nut
cashew	pistachio
chestnut	walnut
coconut	water chestnut
hazelnut	

flax seed
poppu seed
pumpkin seed
sesame seed
sunflower seed
other

SPICES

all spice	cinnamon	galangal	saffron
aniseed	cloves	ginger	turmeric
caraway seed	coriander	grains of paradise	vanilla
cassia	cumin	nettle	*other*
	fenugreek	peppercorn	

HERBS

angelica	fennel	sage	savory
basil	hyssop	mint	sweet cicely
borage	kaffir lime leaves	mustard	sweet woodruff
chervil	lavender	oregano	tarragon

Table 17.2 *(cont'd)*

chives	lemon grass	parsley	thyme
coriander	lemon myrtle	primrose	*other*
cress	lemon verbena	purslane	
dandelion	lovage	rocket	
dill	marjoram	rosemary	

PROCESSED FOODS (including additives – flavourings, colourants, preservatives, etc.)

Table 17.2 Culinary groups

Note: To find a specific food using table 17.2, read aloud (or point to) the major categories, given in capital letters. For any category that produces an indicator change, identify any subcategories in the same way. To narrow down an individual food from a long list, point to each column. You may need to make a distinction between organic and non-organic foods. In the case of fish, you may need to make a distinction between (organically or inorganically) farmed and wild fish.

Protein
Carbohydrate
Fat[1]
Vitamin (use Ridler chart)
Mineral (use Ridler chart)

Table 17.3 Nutritional groups

---

1 *Saturated fats* (mainly animal fats – meat, dairy, eggs) should be limited in the diet. As far as possible *trans-fatty acids* should be avoided since high intake is associated with heart disease. Although dairy products and meat contain small amounts of trans-fatty acids, most consumption derives from commercially prepared baked foods, hard margarine, snacks and other processed foods. Commercially prepared fast foods are also high in trans-fatty acids. Many oils rich in polyunsaturated fats – such as corn oil, sunflower oil, sesame oil and mixed vegetable oil – become unstable when heated and turn into trans-fatty acids. Such oils should only be consumed cool or cold (not cooked). Oils rich in monounsaturated fats, such as olive oil, peanut oil (groundnut oil) and rapeseed oil remain stable when heated and are the oils to use for cooking.

18
Remedies & Supplements

The pendulum provides a reliable means of letting your body choose the remedies and supplements which are good for you, and identifying those which have an adverse effect on your body. The pendulum can help you to make the best choices for your diet, but it is not intended to replace professional advice.

Do you need food supplements? Some authorities argue that, if you're eating the right foods, supplements are unnecessary. But other nutritionists believe that due to (1) increased levels of stress, and (2) depletion of quality of soil combined with use of pesticides and artificial fertilizers which may kill the energy of plants, supplementation is necessary for many people. Even foods labelled 'organic' may be lacking nutritionally (for more on food see chapter 17). On the other hand, many people take supplements that their body doesn't need and are stressful to the body.[1] Some supplements are both detrimental and beneficial – in that there is something in the supplement the body needs, but there is also something in the supplement that is harmful.

You don't necessarily need to take a position about whether supplements are generally required. You can find out whether *you* require them by using the pendulum; you can also identify the *remedies* which will be most beneficial for you; and you can make sure that you are choosing the best supplements and taking them at the right times and in the most appropriate doses.

Also bear in mind that a deficiency may be due to a problem metabolizing the nutrient, rather than a deficiency *per se*. If this is the case, it is better to address the metabolic process rather than simply supplementing the nutrient. Give yourself a balance on the issue of metabolizing the nutrient.

---

1 Intolerance or sensitivity may be to the preparation of the supplement rather than the nutrient itself.

You can find out which remedies or supplements will help you generally; and you can identify the supplements or remedies most beneficial for a specific problem (such as an illness, ailment or emotional difficulty) or goal (such as a sporting event or an important work event).

1☐ *General benefit:* think about everything you're going through at the moment (you don't need to bring all your issues to consciousness: your unconscious body is quite aware of them); the pendulum will give you a signal change. Your subsequent testing will be in relation to what's going on generally in the present.

2☐ *A specific issue:* alternatively, think about a specific problem or goal; the pendulum will give you a signal change. All the testing you now do is in relation to this issue.

Quick testing

When testing a remedy or supplement there are four possibilities:

1☐ The remedy is beneficial (*biogenic*).
2☐ The remedy is detrimental (*biocidic*).
3☐ The remedy is useless but not harmful (*biostatic*).
4☐ The remedy is both beneficial and detrimental; that is, something in it will help, while something else in it will harm (*biogenic* and *biocidic*).

To test, place the container or the tablet/capsule against your navel or on your parotid gland (the cheek). If using IC mode (indicator change mode), for all but number 3 you'll get an indicator change. An indicator change means that the remedy or supplement has some effect. You can verbally ask if it is good for you (or bad for you), or use +/– mode.

A remedy can be both beneficial and detrimental. Use totality mode (see pages 300–1) to see if it is more beneficial or more detrimental overall. Alternatively, you can use priority mode. If you get a signal change when you use priority mode your body is recommending that you take the remedy.

Testing for supplements

There are a few questions you probably want to ask about supplements (such as vitamins and minerals) that you're considering taking:

- *Is this supplement going to help me?*
- *Can it do me any harm?*
- *Is it the best brand for me to take?*
- *What's the best dose for me?*
- *How often should I take it and do I need to take it at any specific times?*
- *How long do I need to take it for?*

Generally speaking, it is preferable, if possible, to obtain your nutrients from eating a good diet rather than taking supplements. Better than simply ascertaining which supplements you need, find out:

- How you can change your diet to render the supplements unnecessary.
- Whether there are blocks to your metabolism that you can resolve with kinesiology techniques.
- Whether there are specific stresses which are burning up your reserves and increasing your requirements for nutrients.

Testing efficacy

The more your body knows about the supplement the better able it is to make any judgement. Bringing the supplement into your aura will give your body a good idea. Consuming it will give your body an even better idea.

But often you will need to make a decision without ingesting it. Whether or not your body is already intimately acquainted with the supplement, place or hold the bottle containing the supplement (or the supplement itself) close to your navel (over clothing is fine). If your body reacts negatively to a plastic bottle (if you suspect this you can simply ask your body), take the supplement out of the container. You can then find out the benefit or otherwise of the substance.

42 CORRECTION
Determining the benefit or detriment of a supplement

1   With the pendulum swinging on the YES–POSITIVE axis, take the supplement container (or the supplement itself) and hold it close to your navel (over clothing is fine).

2   If the pendulum changes its swing to the NO–STRESSED axis, it is probably detrimental to you, but you are going to double check.

3   Switch to indicator change mode (IC mode). Open your palm (the one holding the container or supplement) and let it face upwards. This means YES, and it also means POSITIVE or GOOD FOR YOU.

4   If the pendulum gives a signal change it is good for you or has something which your body needs.

5   Whether the body has indicated that the supplement is good for you or not, turn your palm over so that your knuckles are facing upwards (it doesn't matter whether you are still holding the container to your navel or not; your body knows what you are dealing with). Knuckles upwards means NO and it also means NEGATIVE or DETRIMENTAL TO YOU.

6   If the indicator changes its swing the supplement is bad for you or has ingredients that are harmful or stress your body.

It's commonly the case that a supplement is both beneficial and detrimental. If this is the case you have a choice:

1⊓   You can find another supplement or brand that is good for you and isn't also bad for you (perhaps because it is more natural or doesn't contain other ingredients that harm you).

2⊓   You can determine whether the supplement will do you more good than harm (and vice-versa).

3⊓   You can determine whether this supplement is a priority.

How do you know whether the supplement will do you more good than harm? Apply totality mode.

Totality mode

Totality mode (discovered by the author) enables you to find out the effect of a stimulus on your whole body. If you learn that the supplement is both beneficial and detrimental, apply totality mode (exercise 18.1). Place your thumb pad over the nail of your little finger, and tightly curl up your forefinger against your thumb (see figure 18.1).

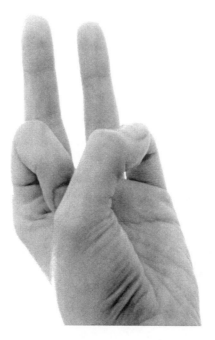

Figure 18.1 Totality mode

Exercise 18.1 Applying totality mode

Note: for this exercise you will either get a signal change with your palm facing up (palm mode) or with the knuckles facing up (knuckles mode); you won't get an indicator change for both.

1 Apply totality mode and palm mode together: hold totality mode with your *palm* facing upwards. If you get a signal change, the supplement is better for you overall than it is detrimental. If you don't get a signal change, go to point 2.
2 Apply totality mode and knuckles mode together: hold totality mode with your *knuckles* facing upwards. If you get a signal change, the supplement is more detrimental for you than it is beneficial and should be avoided.

Brand testing

If you are in a shop, you can test several brands of the same supplement. If your body indicates that it needs the supplement, you can find the best one for you (which will not necessarily be the best for anyone else) by using priority mode (exercise 18.2).

Exercise 18.2 Testing for the best brand

1   Pick up the first supplement container and hold it close to your navel (or your cheek).
2   Apply totality mode with palm mode. If you get a signal change the supplement will do you more good than harm.
3   Test several supplements in the same way.
4   Retest each supplement that produced a signal change using priority mode (tip of middle finger to inside middle crease of thumb). Have in mind that you want the *highest priority* supplement (of those tested) to indicate.
5   The supplement that produces a signal change is the best one for you at this time.

Some people 'test' products in their imagination that they have no direct experience of – varieties found on the internet, for example. Your body will certainly give you an answer if you ask it for the best one that you can find on the web. But the answer won't be very reliable, since it is making the decision on very limited information. The more information the body has, the more reliable the judgement. It will have the best information on products you have consumed. Otherwise, bringing substances into your aura and holding them close to the navel is generally agreed to be pretty reliable.

Dosage

It's best to establish your dose after you have ingested a small amount of the supplement, since your body then has better information.

Exercise 18.3 Dosage

Before you begin this exercise first check the recommended daily dose. Don't exceed any maximum stated dose. Using the pendulum you will find out the quantity of the dose; then you will establish the number of doses.

1   If the supplement comes in tablet or capsule form, take one out of the container and put it on the lid. If it is in liquid form, put a spoonful, or whatever measurement you're using, in a glass and hold that to the navel.[1]

2   Have the pendulum swinging, and pick up the lid with the tablet or capsule (or a glass containing a measurement of the liquid supplement) and put it next to your navel.

3   If you get an indicator change (which you will, if you need the supplement), put a second tablet or capsule on the lid (or a second measurement in the glass) and hold it next to your navel.

4   Repeat until you do not get an indicator change. You now have one too many, so put one tablet or capsule back, and you have your dose. (If you're putting spoonfuls, for example, in a glass, make sure you remember how many you've put in. Subtract one spoonful, and you have your dose.)

You know your dose. But how many doses per day? Don't exceed any stated maximum number. Ask: *At least once a day? At least twice a day?* – until you no longer get an indicator change. If, for example, the pendulum stopped giving an indicator change on *At least four times a day?* then the supplement is required three times a day.

If the dose is less than one a day, find out how many doses per week. Ask: *At least one a week? At least two a week?* – until you no longer get an indicator change. If, for example, the pendulum stopped giving an indicator change on *At least five a week?* then the supplement is required four times a week. If this is the case, find out which days to take it. It may be every other day; or working days; or whatever. Trust your intuition and confirm with the pendulum.

---

1   Kinesiologists generally place substances to be tested close to the navel because this area is a major junction for energy circuits.

To find out the optimum times to take the supplement, say: *It matters what time I take them.* If you get a YES (as you probably will), ask: *Is it activity time?* If no, ask: *Is it clock time?* If it's *activity time* it will probably be before, during or after a meal (but could relate to a different activity, of course, such as going to bed, or exercise, or work). Ask to find out. If it's *clock time*, determine the times of day. You might need, instead, to find out when *not* to take it.

Finding out how long to take the supplement for is also straightforward. Find out whether your unit of measurement should be days, weeks or months. Then ask: *I need to take this for at least one day/week/month; At least two days/weeks/months* – and so on, until you get no indicator change (which means that's one day, week or month too long). Remember that your body is making a prediction from what it knows today. It could change its mind. Towards the end of this period, ask your body again.

Bach remedies

Bach flower remedies[1] are well known and widely available. If you possess the remedies you can test using the remedies themselves (the procedure is outlined below). The principles outlined here are the same for any remedies. If you don't possess any remedies, it can still be helpful to find out which (conscious or unconscious) mood(s) to address by using the written categories of the Bach flower remedies (see below). Recognizing and acknowledging the emotions and moods brings them on line and ready for resolution.

The finger mode for essences such as Bach is on the emotional finger: place the thumb pad over the nail of the ring finger (figure 18.2).

Testing with written categories

You can test with written categories even if you don't have the remedies (# 43a). If you have them, you might prefer to use the remedies themselves for the testing (# 43b).

---

1   A medical doctor, Edward Bach, gave up his work in general practice in 1930 to pursue natural remedies. Led by his intuition, he discovered plants which healed his moods. He died in 1936, aged 50, having discovered 38 flower essences which he considered to be a complete system.

After testing, if you have the remedies, you can mix a composite remedy. If you don't have the remedies, the exercise is still very helpful: it will enable you to identify your conscious and unconscious (and perhaps repressed) feelings and moods – so you can acknowledge and resolve them. I suggest that you either (1) do a full balance and check the moods again afterwards; or (2) do F/O holding (# 9, page 98) and bring your attention to your body as you acknowledge the feelings and moods that indicated and consider how they apply to you in the present. EFT could also be useful.

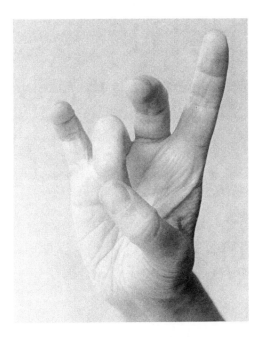

Figure 18.2 Essence finger mode

43a CORRECTION
Balancing with Bach remedies (categories)

1   Either (a) put your attention on what's generally going on for you right now; (b) think about a specific issue; or (c) state your goal. As the pendulum gives you an indicator change to register this, put it into circuit (put legs apart).
2   Using table 18.1 (page 307), name each major category (*fear, uncertainty* and so on). For each one that gives a signal change, go through the list of moods/remedies and take a note of all that indicate.

3   If you get more than seven[1] ask your body to help you to reduce the
        number to seven or fewer by indicating the moods/remedies that are
        not a priority. State each of the moods/remedies that indicated again
        and the ones that indicate now can be discarded.
4   While doing frontal/occipital holding (which you can put into circuit
        if preferred), read the information about each remedy from Edward
        Bach's descriptions (pages 308–13). If possible, acknowledge how these
        apply to you in the present.
5   If you have the remedies, prepare the composite remedy;[2] if you don't,
        take a SUD score and give yourself a balance (or more ESR or some
        EFT).

Testing with Bach remedies themselves

If you possess the Bach remedies, instead of using the written categories you
can test with the bottles themselves. The laborious way of doing this would
be to test each bottle separately by placing them, one at a time, on the navel
and seeing their effect on the pendulum. But there are 38 bottles, and it's
quicker to test a few at a time.

43b CORRECTION
Balancing with Bach remedies (bottles)

1   Either (a) put your attention on what's generally going on for you right
        now; (b) think about a specific issue; or (c) state your goal. As the pendu-
        lum gives you a signal change to register this, put it into circuit (put
        legs apart).
2   Touch four bottles at once, using one finger for each bottle. (It is prefer-
        able to touch the bottles themselves rather than the bottle caps.) If
        you get an indicator change, touch two of the four bottles. If you get an

---

1   Using more than seven remedies is confusing to the body and should be
avoided.

2   Place two drops from each bottle into a mixer bottle containing fresh mineral or spring water. Gently shake the bottle. Add four drops of this solution to
a drink of water (or other liquid), or take directly on to the tongue. The remedy
should be taken first thing in the morning, last thing at night, and as often as
you want during the day (but a *minimum* of four times). You cannot overdose
and it can't do you any harm.

Category	Remedy	Mood
Fear	Aspen	Foreboding; unknown fears
	Cherry plum	Strong temper; fear of doing harm
	Mimulus	Shyness; timidity; fear of known things;
	Red chestnut	Over-concern for the welfare of loved ones
	Rock rose	Panic, terror; extreme fright
Uncertainty	Cerato	Doubts own judegment
	Gentian	Easily discouraged, dejected
	Gorse	Extreme hopelessness; despair
	Hornbeam	Monday morning feeling; procrastination
	Scieranthus	Uncertainty; indecision; mood swings
	Wild oat	Unfulfilled; ambitions unclear
Lack of interest in present circumstances	Clematis	Day-dreaming; indifference; inattention
	Chestnut bud	Repeats mistakes
	Honeysuckle	Fixed on the past; homesick
	Mustard	Deep gloom; melancholia
	Olive	Complete exhaustion
	White chestnut	Persistent, unwanted thoughts
	Wild rose	Resignation; apathy; lack of ambition
Loneliness	Heather	Self-absorbed, dislike of being alone
	Impatiens	Impatient; hasty; easily irritated
	Water violet	Proud, reserved; aloof
Oversensitivity to influence of others	Agrimony	Cheerful face hiding inner torture
	Centaury	Can't say no; eager to please; trampled on
	Holly	Envy; jealousy; lack of love for others
	Walnut	Going through major life changes; in need of protection from influence of others

Table 18.1 Bach remedy categories

indicator change, find out which one or whether both of the bottles are indicated. Then check the other two bottles in the same way. Put any indicated bottles to the side.

3   Keep testing in batches of four until you have tested all the bottles.

4   If more than seven bottles are indicated ask your body to help you to reduce the number to seven or fewer by indicating the moods/ remedies that are *not* a priority. Place each of the previously indicated remedies on the body and the ones that now give a signal change can be discarded.

5   While doing frontal/occipital holding (which you can put into circuit if preferred), read the detailed information about each indicated priority remedy from Edward Bach's descriptions below. If possible, acknowledge how these apply to you in the present.

6   Mix up a composite remedy by putting two drops of each indicated remedy into a bottle with fresh mineral or spring water. Shake the bottle gently and add four drops to a drink of water (or other liquid) first thing in the morning, last thing at night, and as frequently as desired during the day.

The descriptions under each remedy (which come from *The Twelve Healers and Other Remedies*, by Edward Bach) do not necessarily describe your personality (although they may do so); they may describe your mood in the present, or an aspect of your mood, or be specifically related just to the issue you are working with. The advantage of identifying the remedies with the pendulum is that characteristics present themselves that you may deny or disavow consciously. *Pay even greater attention to disavowed characteristics.* By identifying disavowed characteristics the pendulum (like muscle testing) makes using such remedies even more powerful than when they are consciously identified.

The 38 remedies in Edward Bach's own words:[1]

Agrimony
The jovial, cheerful, humorous people who love peace and are distressed by argument or quarrel, to avoid which they will agree to give up much. Though generally they have troubles and are tormented and restless and worried in mind or in body, they hide their cares behind their humour and jesting and are considered very good friends to know. They often take alcohol or drugs in excess, to stimulate themselves and help themselves bear their trials with cheerfulness.

Aspen
Vague unknown fears, for which there can be given no explanation, no reason. Yet the patient may be terrified of something terrible going to happen, he knows not what. These vague unexplainable fears may haunt by night or day. Sufferers often are afraid to tell their trouble to others.

1   An excellent book on using the Bach remedies is *Bach* by Pat, available from Pat Herington: pat@herington.plus.com.

Beech

For those who feel the need to see more good and beauty in all that surrounds them. And, although much appears to be wrong, to have the ability to see the good growing within. So as to be able to be more tolerant, lenient and understanding of the different way each individual and all things are working to their own final perfection.

Centaury

Kind, quiet, gentle people who are over-anxious to serve others. They overtax their strength in their endeavours. Their wish so grows upon them that they become more servants than willing helpers. Their good nature leads them to do more than their own share of work, and in so doing they may neglect their own particular mission in life.

Cerato

Those who have not sufficient confidence in themselves to make their own decisions. They constantly seek advice from others, and are often misguided.

Cherry plum

Fear of the mind being over-strained, of reason giving way, of doing fearful and dreaded things, not wished and known wrong, yet there comes the thought and impulse to do them.

Chestnut bud

For those who do not take full advantage of observation and experience, and who take a longer time than others to learn the lessons of daily life. Whereas one experience would be enough for some, such people find it necessary to have more, sometimes several, before the lesson is learnt. Therefore, to their regret, they find themselves having to make the same error on different occasions when once would have been enough, or observation of others could have spared them even that one fault.

Chicory

Those who are very mindful of the needs of others; they tend to be over-full of care for children, relatives, friends, always finding something that should be put right. They are continually correcting what they consider wrong, and enjoy doing so. They desire that those for whom they care should be near them.

Clematis

Those who are dreamy, drowsy, not fully awake, no great interest in life. Quiet people, not really happy in their present circumstances, living more in the future than in the present; living in hopes of happier times, when their ideals may come true. In illness some make little or no effort to get well, and in certain cases may even look forward to death, in the hope of better times; or maybe, meeting again some beloved one whom they have lost.

Crab apple

'This is the remedy of cleansing. For those who feel as if they had something not quite clean about themselves. Often it is something of apparently little importance: in others there may be more serious disease which is almost disregarded compared to the one thing on which they concentrate. In both types they are anxious to be free from the one particular thing which is greatest in their minds and which seems so essential to them that it should be cured. They become despondent if treatment fails. Being a cleanser, this remedy purifies wounds if the patient has reason to believe that some poison has entered which must be drawn out.'

Elm

'Those who are doing good work, are following the calling of their life and who hope to do something of importance, and this often for the benefit of humanity. At times there may be periods of depression when they feel that the task they have undertaken is too difficult, and not within the power of a human being.'

Gentian

'Those who are easily discouraged. They may be progressing well in illness, or in the affairs of their daily life, but any small delay or hindrance to progress causes doubt and soon disheartens them.'

Gorse

'Very great hopelessness, they have given up belief that more can be done for them. Under persuasion or to please others they may try different treatments, at the same time assuring those around that there is so little hope of relief.'

Heather

'Those who are always seeking the companionship of anyone who may be available, as they find it necessary to discuss their own affairs with others, no matter whom it may be. They are very unhappy if they have to be alone for any length of time.'

Holly

'For those who sometimes are attacked by thoughts of such kind as jealousy, envy, revenge, suspicion. For the different forms of vexation. Within themselves they may suffer much, often when there is no real cause for their unhappiness.'

Honeysuckle

'Those who live much in the past, perhaps a time of great happiness, or memories of a lost friend, or ambitions which have not come true. They do not expect further happiness such as they have had.'

Hornbeam

'For those who feel that they have not sufficient strength, mentally or physically, to carry the burden of life placed upon them; the affairs of every day seem too much for them to accomplish, though they generally succeed in fulfilling their task. For those who believe that some part, of mind or body, needs to be strengthened before they can easily fulfil their work.'

Impatiens

'Those who are quick in thought and action and who wish all things to be done without hesitation or delay. When ill they are anxious for a hasty recovery. They find it very difficult to be patient with people who are slow, as they consider it wrong and a waste of time, and they will endeavour to make such people quicker in all ways. They often prefer to work and think alone, so that they can do everything at their own speed.'

Larch

'For those who do not consider themselves as good or capable as those around them, who expect failure, who feel that they will never be a success, and so do not venture or make a strong enough attempt to succeed.'

Mimulus

'Fear of worldly things, illness, pain, accidents, poverty, of dark, of being alone, of misfortune. The fears of everyday life. These people quietly and secretly bear their dread, they do not freely speak of it to others.'

Mustard

'Those who are liable to times of gloom, or even despair, as though a cold dark cloud overshadowed them and hid the light and the joy of life. It may not be possible to give any reason or explanation for such attacks. Under these conditions it is almost impossible to appear happy or cheerful.'

Oak

'For those who are struggling and fighting strongly to get well, or in connection with the affairs of their daily life. They will go on trying one thing after another, though their case may seem hopeless. They will fight on. They are discontented with themselves if illness interferes with their duties or helping others. They are brave people, fighting against great difficulties, without loss of hope or effort.'

Olive

'Those who have suffered much mentally or physically and are so exhausted and weary that they feel they have no more strength to make any effort. Daily life is hard work for them, without pleasure.'

Pine

'For those who blame themselves. Even when successful they think that they could have done better, and are never content with their efforts or the results. They are hard working and suffer much from the faults they attach to themselves. Sometimes if there is any mistake it is due to another, but they will claim responsibility even for that.'

Red chestnut

'For those who find it difficult not to be anxious for other people. Often they have ceased to worry about themselves, but for those of whom they are fond they may suffer much, frequently anticipating that some unfortunate thing may happen to them.'

Rock rose

'The rescue remedy. The remedy of emergency for cases where there even appears no hope. In accident or sudden illness, or when the patient is very frightened or terrified or if the condition is serious enough to cause great fear to those around. If the patient is not conscious the lips may be moistened with the remedy.'

Rock water

'Those who are very strict in their way of living; they deny themselves many of the joys and pleasures of life because they consider it might interfere with their work. They are hard masters to themselves. They wish to be well and strong and active, and will do anything which they believe will keep them so. They hope to be examples which will appeal to others who may then follow their ideas and be better as a result.'

Scleranthus

'Those who suffer much from being unable to decide between two things, first one seeming right then the other. They are usually quiet people, and bear their difficulty alone, as they are not inclined to discuss it with others.'

Star of Bethlehem

'For those in great distress under conditions which for a time produce great unhappiness. The shock of serious news, the loss of someone dear, the fright following an accident, and such like. For those who for a time refuse to be consoled this remedy brings comfort.'

Sweet chestnut

'For those moments which happen to some people when the anguish is so great as to seem to be unbearable. When the mind or body feels as if it had borne to the uttermost limit of its endurance, and that now it must give way. When it seems there is nothing but destruction and annihilation left to face.'

Vervain

'Those with fixed principles and ideas, which they are confident are right, and which they very rarely change. They have a great wish to convert all around them to their own views of life. They are strong of will and have much courage when they are convinced of those things that they wish to teach. In illness they struggle on long after many would have given up their duties.'

Vine

'Very capable people, certain of their own ability, confident of success. Being so assured, they think that it would be for the benefit of others if they could be persuaded to do things as they themselves do, or as they are certain is right. Even in illness they will direct their attendants. They may be of great value in emergency.'

Walnut

'For those who have definite ideals and ambitions in life and are fulfilling them, but on rare occasions are tempted to be led away from their own ideas, aims and work by the enthusiasm, convictions or strong opinions of others. The remedy gives constancy and protection from outside influences.'

Water violet

'For those who in health or illness like to be alone. Very quiet people, who move about without noise, speak little, and then gently. Very independent, capable and self-reliant. Almost free of the opinions of others. They are aloof, leave people alone and go their own way. Often clever and talented. Their peace and calmness is a blessing to those around them.'

White chestnut

'For those who cannot prevent thoughts, ideas, arguments which they do not desire from entering their minds. Usually at such times when the interest of the moment is not strong enough to keep the mind full. Thoughts which worry and will remain, or if for a time thrown out, will return. They seem to circle round and round and cause mental torture. The presence of such unpleasant thoughts drives out peace and interferes with being able to think only of the work or pleasure of the day.'

Wild oat

'Those who have ambitions to do something of prominence in life, who wish to have much experience, and to enjoy all that which is possible for them, to take life to the full. Their difficulty is to determine what occupation to follow; as although their ambitions are strong, they have no calling which appeals to them above all others. This may cause delay and dissatisfaction.'

Wild rose

'Those who without apparently sufficient reason become resigned to all that happens, and just glide through life, take it as it is, without any effort to improve things and find some joy. They have surrendered to the struggle of life without complaint.'

Willow

'For those who have suffered adversity or misfortune and find these difficult to accept, without complaint or resentment, as they judge life much by the success which it brings. They feel that they have not deserved so great a trial, that it was unjust, and they become embittered. They often take less interest and less activity in those things of life which they had previously enjoyed.'

19
A New Beginning

You have made significant progress in learning an invaluable skill which you can use for any number of problems, goals and other purposes. Unlike most people who use the pendulum or some other method of dowsing, you know that, when you use the pre-tests and the pendulum mode, your results are highly likely to be accurate and reliable. However, you are aware of the pendulum's limitations and know that it does not give God's Truth.

You have an extensive range of kinesiology corrections and energy therapy techniques which will help you to heal past issues, achieve goals, develop your intuition, and restore and maintain good health and a sense of well-being. On a daily basis you can test for supplements, check your diet, test for food sensitivities, and free yourself of unnecessary emotional baggage.With practice and experience, you can also successfully resolve longstanding and deep-seated emotional problems.

There are many ways of using the material in this book. Mastering the techniques and giving yourself full balances with respect to specific issues and goals would help you to become a first-rate self-therapist. But you can use the material in many other ways. I'd like to encourage you to explore this material and find what works best for you. Adapt my suggestions. Incorporate other corrections or methods that you know about or come across which are useful to you.

Here are some ideas:

- ○ Just do the corrections and exercises as you read and re-read the book, or while focusing on your issues. This is greatly beneficial to your health and well-being.

○ Any time you have a few moments to spare, use the pendulum to find out which single correction would be most helpful right now (appendix 3).

○ If there are corrections you haven't yet managed to get the hang of, leave them out. Your corrections repertoire can include just the corrections you specify. (You don't have to do it 'by the book', do it all, or get it all right – do you? If you feel you do, you may want to choose to become more flexible in your attitude.)

○ In addition to full balances (including problem and goal) you can perform instant mini-balances with regard to specific problems, by limiting your application of corrections to the present time (that is, without going back to the sources of the issue).

○ Address an issue in the present just using alarm points and the energy corrections (including lymphatic and vascular reflexes and any other corrections you want to include from chapter 10).

○ Go back to the source of an issue and address the issue using alarm points and energy corrections from chapter 10. This is a great way of doing a quick balance.

○ Give yourself a time of day balance, in the present, with (or without) an issue or goal.

○ Give yourself a balance using only the correction(s) that you know well or can remember without looking up.

○ Determine the optimum food or nutrients for a specific goal.

○ Use the chart adapted from Dr Ridler to determine any nutritional deficiencies.

○ Address any problem just using EFT. Many therapists only use EFT in their practice. You can do even better: go to the source of the issue and apply EFT there.

○ Use the pendulum to find the sources of any problem.

Remember that it's important to find the priority problem, as well as the priority remedy. This will make your efforts far more efficient and economical.

Don't put this book away on the shelf. This is just the beginning of your journey. Take the time to apply these methods to your issues. Use this volume as a reference manual. It contains a wealth of powerful material for your personal health and development (but of course sometimes the help of a good therapist may be helpful or necessary). Undertake to use these methods regularly. Why not address one past issue each week? When bad feelings, issues and problems come up, pick up your pendulum and find the best way to resolve them.

Use the protocol in the appendix, or simply put the issue in circuit and find the priority correction. Remember to take SUD and VOC readings to measure your progress. Keep a check on your overall health and well-being by taking an audit of your life indexes (table 11.1, page 185).

Don't forget that your unconscious body is not infallible or all-knowing. The messages of your unconscious via the pendulum will sometimes be contradictory; sometimes your unconscious will seem to change its mind; or, rather than taking a straight route, you may seem to meander or backtrack as you progress through an issue. You might also have responses that don't seem to make sense. This is all to be expected. It doesn't mean it's not working or that you should give up.

Stay with it. Trust your unconscious. It wants to help and it's doing its best to help you. All it needs is a good opportunity. Sometimes it may not know how to tell you something, or has to tell you in a very roundabout or peculiar way involving a number of different stages that you don't at first understand. Let your body find a way to give you effective help. Your initial question, issue or approach may not give it the best opportunity to express what it wants directly, but it will do its best to find a way of telling you what you need to know.

Regularly tune in to your unconscious body, since doing so is the most effective way of staying happy and congruent. Attend to your feelings. Use your intuition as well as the pendulum to maintain this contact. Trust and respect your body. When the choice is between heart and head, choose heart: in other words, choose what you *feel* is best for you, not what you *think* is best. Your feelings are nearly always right, even when they're wrong – and it's fine to be wrong; it's the best way to learn. It's better to be wrong for the right reasons than right for the wrong reasons. The wisdom of your body is based on your experiences. Judgement based on your experience is the best judgement you've got. Believe and trust your intuition. The more in touch you are with your unconscious body, the less you'll need the pendulum.

Notice the changes that you make in the way you feel, think and behave, in your beliefs about yourself and the world, and in your health. Give appreciation to your body for helping you to make these changes. Remain humble and give appreciation to your unconscious body, and everything and everyone that has helped you, when you make progress.

Keep setting yourself new goals. Accept that all worthwhile goals involve challenges. Meet these challenges and resolve the issues that emerge as you move towards achieving your goals. Whatever happens, keep going forward.

APPENDICES

APPENDIX 1
Pre-checks

Pre-test # 1
Central meridian over-energy

1☐　Start with the pendulum swinging on your YES axis.

2☐　Zip up the central meridian. If there is an indicator change, make the correction.

3☐　Zip down the central meridian. If there is *no* indicator change make the correction.

4☐　To correct: EITHER: *flush* by zipping up and down the meridian; OR: use the harmonizing posture.

Pre-test # 2
Hydration

1☐　To check for hydration, say: *Water*.

2☐　If there is an indicator change, drink (sipping, not gulping) a glass of water (preferably not tap water) and recheck.

Pre-test # 3
Left–right switching

1☐　Hold the K27s with a neutral touch. If there is an indicator change, make the correction.

2☐　To correct: place one hand over the navel and with the other massage both K27s. Swap hands and repeat.

Pre-test # 4
Up–down switching

1☐   Hold the ends of the central and governing meridians (just below the middle of your bottom lip and under nose) with a neutral touch. If there is an indicator change, make the correction.

2☐   To correct: place one hand over the navel and, with the other, massage both points (under nose and below bottom lip) simultaneously. Swap hands and repeat.

Pre-test # 5
Forward–backward switching

1☐   Hold the end of the coccyx. If there is an indicator change, make the correction.

2☐   To correct: place one hand over the navel and, with the other, massage the end of the coccyx. Swap hands and repeat.

Pre-test # 6
Balanced ionization

1☐   Block one nostril with a neutral touch and breathe in through the open nostril. Check for an indicator change.

2☐   Breathe out through the same nostril. Again, check for a signal change.

3☐   Do the same with the other nostril.

4☐   If any breath produced a signal change, make the correction.

5☐   To correct, breathe in through one nostril and out through the other.

6☐   Then change: breathe in through the nostril you breathed out of and out through the in nostril.

7☐   Repeat until this individual nostril breathing does not produce an indicator change.

Pre-test # 7
Hyperstress

1☐ Using IC mode (and palm mode), say: *My body is receptive and amenable to change.* If you get an indicator change, you're fine. If you don't, your body is probably in hyperstress. Do the correction.

2☐ Still holding the pendulum with one hand, place your other hand over you forehead very gently, touching your frontal eminences (the two bumps, prominent in some people, on the forehead between the eyebrows and the hairline) but without applying any pressure.

3☐ Relax and breathe. Keep your hand on your forehead until you get a signal change telling you that the hyperstress is corrected.

Remember, simply performing the pre-tests can help calm you and improve your energy.

APPENDIX 2
The Steps of the Full Self-kinesiology Balance

1   Do the pre-checks and ask permission to address your issue.

2   Use the pendulum to find and confirm the best wording for your goal.

3   *Optional:* Find the percentage of stress involved and the available energy to address the issue.

4   *Optional:* Identify and acknowledge the primary emotion(s).

5   Ask: *Do I need more information?* If you do, find out what.

6   Ask: *Am I ready to correct?* If not, find out if you need more information or check that you have permission. Trust whatever comes up.

7   Ask: *Are there any corrections to be done in present time?* If so, ask: *Do I need a meridian?* If you need a meridian, use the alarm points to find the priority meridian and the correction(s) required. Perform the correction(s) for the meridian.

8   Ask: *Are there any more corrections in the present?* If so, identify and perform the correction(s).

9   Ask: *Do I have permission to go back in time?* If the answer is no, do F/O holding while thinking through the issue. You can also ask what else you need to do first.

10   Once you have permission, go back to the antecedent age. When you reach this age, establish what was happening. If this proves very difficult, ask whether it is necessary to know consciously what was happening. If it is, keep eliciting information until the pendulum agrees that you have all the information you need.

11   *Optional:* Identify the primary emotion(s) and the percentage stressors and available energy at this specific age.

12   Ask: *Am I ready to correct this?* If not, find out if you need more information, or if something else is required. When you're ready to correct,

ask if you need a meridian, and find it using the alarm points. Correct the meridians in priority order. Then find out what other corrections are required and perform them.

13   *Optional:* Check that the emotion from number 11 above is now clear by restating the emotion. If it is now clear, there will be no signal change. Also re-check the percentage of stressors and available energy pertinent to this age.

14   *Optional:* Ask: *Are there other ages to visit?* If so, ask: *Backward in time?* If yes, go backwards in time. If no, ask: *Forward in time?* If yes, go forward in time. When you get to the next antecedent age, find out all the information required. Then proceed from number 11 above.

15   Ask permission to return to the present, and ask the pendulum to give you a signal change when you're fully back in the present.

16   *Optional:* Recheck the original primary emotion. It should now be clear. Also recheck percentage of stressors (which should have changed and may be at zero) and available energy (which should have changed and may be at 100).

17   Ask: *Do I have permission to visit the goal?* If granted, imagine you have now achieved your goal. Using the present tense, describe what it means to you to have achieved it. When you are ready, check with the pendulum that your visit to the goal is complete. Ask permission to return to the present, and for an indicator change when you're there.

18   In the present, restate your goal. If there's an indicator change you know there's more work to be done.

19   Ask: *Is there more work to be done on this issue?* If so, find out when you can come back to it.

20   Finally, thank your body for the work it has done and the changes it has made. Undertake to be responsible for making it happen.

APPENDIX 3
Directory of Methods, Tests & Corrections

Note: not all the corrections have a specific test; or the test is taken as part of the correction.

		Test	Correction
# 1	Auditory perception	66	66
# 2	Visual perception	68	69
# 3	Brain integration (cross-crawl)	78	78
# 4	Brain integration (cross-crawl) with eye movements	–	81
# 5	Tracing the lemniscate for vision	–	82
# 6	Tracing the lemniscate for writing	–	84
# 7	Gait reflexes	84	85
# 8	Emotional stress release (ESR)	91	91
# 9	Frontal–occipital holding	–	98
# 10	Emotional distress release (EDR)	–	99
# 11	Colour balance	–	101
# 12	Acknowledging the involved emotion		126
# 13	Identifying the antecedents of an issue	–	131
# 14	Neuro-lymphatic (NL) reflexes	154	157
# 15	Neuro-vascular (NV) reflexes	161	161
# 16	Tracing the meridian	–	163
# 17	Acupoints to tonify and sedate	–	164
# 18	Central & governing hook up	–	171
# 19	Time of day balance	–	173
# 20	Balancing acupoints	–	174
# 21	Tracing a meridian backwards to alleviate pain	–	177

Table A3.1 Methods, tests & corrections by number

Table A3.2 Methods, tests & corrections by category

#	Electrical	TEST	CORRECTION
1	Auditory perception	66	66
2	Visual perception	68	69
3	Brain integration (cross-crawl)	78	78
4	Brain integration (cross-crawl) with eye movements	–	81
5	Tracing the lemniscate (vision)	–	82
6	Tracing the lemniscate (writing)	–	84
7	Gait reflexes	84	85
16	Tracing the meridian	–	163
17	Acupoints to tonify and sedate	–	164
18	Central & governing hook-up	–	171
19	Time of day balance	–	173
20	Balancing acupoints	–	174
21	Tracing a meridian backwards (for pain)	–	177
26	Body polarity	232	233
31	Cloacal energy	244	244

#	Emotional	TEST	CORRECTION
8	Emotional stress release (ESR)	91	91
9	Frontal/Occipital holding	–	98
10	Emotional Distress Release (EDR)	–	99
11	Colour balance	–	101
12	Acknowledging the involved emotion	–	126
15	Neuro-vascular (NV) reflexes	161	161
33	Emotional rigidity	248	248
43a	Balancing with Bach remedies (categories)	–	305
43b	Balancing with Bach remedies (bottles)	–	306

#	Biochemical	TEST	CORRECTION
14	Neuro-lymphatic (NL) reflexes	154	157
29	Adrenal stress	237	238
32	RNA/DNA	245	246
37	Environmental allergies & sensitivities	–	274
38	Food compatibility	–	283
39	Identifying food issues	–	286
40a	Identifying nutritional *deficiencies*	–	290
40b	Identifying nutritional *excesses*	–	290
41	Storage, preparation & eating	–	291
42	Benefits/detriments of a supplement	–	300

#	Structural	TEST	CORRECTION
27	Common integrative area	233	234
28	Fixation	236	236
30	Constricted cranials	240	240
35	Ileocecal & Houston valve imbalance	251	252

#	Other methods	TEST	CORRECTION
13	Identifying the antecedents of an issue	–	131
22	Working with life choices	–	186
23	Modelling a third-person perspective	–	186
24	Generating a support system	–	189
25	Giving the problem back (1)	–	197
34	Giving the problem back (2)	–	249
36	Applying EFT	–	264

Note:

Form the digital finger modes one at a time (page 223). An indicator change means that a correction from this category is required. Go down the list, using the correction numbers or stating the name of the correction to find the required correction.

Further Reading

Barhydt, Elizabeth and Barhydt, Hamilton, *Self Help for Stress and Pain* (Loving Life Corporation, 1997)

------, *Accurate Muscle Testing for Foods and Supplements* (Loving Life Corporation, 1992)

Bradshaw, John, *Homecoming: Reclaiming and championing your inner child* (Piatkus Books, 1991)

Diamond, John, *Your Body Doesn't Lie: Introduction to behavioural kinesiology* (Eden Grove Editions, 1997)

Eden, Donna, *Energy Medicine: How to use your body's energies for optimum health and vitality* (Piatkus Books, 2003)

Feinstein, David, Eden, Donna and Craig, Gary, *The Healing Power of EFT and Energy Psychology: Revolutionary methods for dramatic personal change* (Piatkus Books, 2006)

Frost, Robert, *Applied Kinesiology: A training manual and reference book of basic principles* (North Atlantic Books, 2002)

Gendlin, Eugene T., *Focusing* (Bantam Books, 1981)

Holford, Patrick, *Optimum Nutrition Bible* (Piatkus Books, 2004)

Holdway, Ann, *The Wisdom Within: Life enhancing kinesiology* (Ann Holdway, 2008)

Kaptchuck, Ted, J., *The Web that Has No Weaver* (Congdon & Weed, 1982)

Krebs, Charles & Brown, Jenny, *A Revolutionary Way of Thinking* (Hill of Content, 1998)

La Tourelle, Maggie, *Principles of Kinesiology* (Thorsons, 1997)

Promislow, Sharon, *Making the Brain–Body Connection* (Access Publishers Network, 1999)

Thie, John and Thie, Matthew, *Touch for Health: The complete edition* (De Vorss & Co, 2006)

------, *Touch for Health Pocketbook with Chinese 5 Element Metaphors* (Touch for Health Education, 2002)

Topping, Wayne, *Stress Release* (Topping International Institute, 1985)

------, *Success Over Distress* (Topping International Institute, 1990)

Kinesiology
Training & Resources

Touch for Health (the foundation of virtually all the energy kinesiologies) and Three In One Concepts are just two of the many kinesiology systems in which you can train. Although they provide the best tools for my practice, that doesn't necessarily mean they are the best for you. If you are interested in pursuing kinesiology training, I recommend you explore the various options and receive a treatment or balance from a qualified practitioner.

UK

Touch for Health

Sandy Gannon, President of the International Kinesiology College (IKC), and head of Touch for Health in the UK. Email SGannon11@aol.com; www.touch4healthkinesiology.co.uk.

The Touch for Health Centre, Bognor Regis: trustees can be contacted at PO Box 150, Bognor Regis, West Sussex, PO21 2FN. Emails: theruddles@talktalk.net; susanspencer@care4free.net.

Three In One Concepts

Daphne Clarke (England): email DaphneRoberta@gmail.com.

Claire Tomlins (Scotland): email Claire@HarmonyKinesiology.com; or go to www.HarmonyKinesiology.com.

Other Kinesiologies

The Kinesiology Federation is the UK's largest umbrella organization for kinesiologists. Website: www.kinesiologyfederation.org.

United States

Touch for Health

Matthew Thie, Head of Touch for Health Education and Director of Research for the International Kinesiology College. Matthew Thie carries the Touch for Health torch following the founder of TFH, his father, the late Dr John F. Thie. Website: www.touch4health.com.

Three In One Concepts

The President of Three In One Concepts is Anastazya Wada. Email info@3in1concepts.us; and see www.3in1concepts.us. The schedule of Daniel Whiteside, the surviving co-founder of Three In One Concepts, is available from the website.

Electronic

Earl and Gail Cook have spent many years creating a comprehensive source of Touch for Health materials in electronic form. In 2007 they released the second version of ETouch for Health (Touch for Health tools in electronic form). It is a very useful resource. For information and to purchase go to www.etouchforhealth.com.

International

The International Kinesiology College has been the guardian of the Touch for Health synthesis since 1990. Website: www.ikc-info.org.

Meet the author

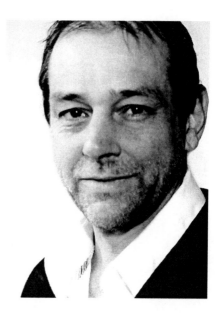

Since opening his practice in 1998, Jonathan Livingstone has been developing and refining the most effective contemporary therapy and coaching methods available. He created Temporal Modelling to identify the sources of problems and Younger Self Resolution to resolve past issues. He is a Touch for Health instructor and an NLP Master Practitioner from NLPU, CA. From 2002 to 2004 he served on the board of the Kinesiology Federation.

He has practices in Leamington Spa and central London and works with organizations as well as individuals, children and couples. He also offers supervision to practitioners and training to professionals and lay people. For information or an appointment, call 07862 226143.

More information is available from: www.TherapyCoaching.co.uk.

He is married to Elizabeth King, principal of development and training at Elysia (UK distributors of Dr.Hauschka skin care), and has two grown-up sons and a daughter, Abigail, born September 2007.

For training in Touch for Health, self-kinesiology with the pendulum, or any of Jonathan's other courses, email jonathan@TherapyCoaching.co.uk.

Comments about your experience with the material in this book are very welcome: email jonathan@TherapistWithin.com.

Lightning Source UK Ltd.
Milton Keynes UK
18 February 2010

150310UK00004B/2/P